How to Perfe Pregnant

by

Pamela Smith, Registered Dietitian

and

Carolyn Coats

Cover by Jodi Coats Burson
Illustrations by Sheila Behr

Thomas Nelson Publishers - Nashville

MW00809098

Table of Contents

Introduction ... 1
The Ten Commandments of Good Nutrition ... 3
Commandment I - Never Skip Breakfast ... 5
The 7 Health Habits for a Longer Life ... 9
Commandment II - Eat Often, Snacks Are Smart! ... 10
Power Snack List ... 13
Commandment III - The Carbo and Protein Balance ... 15
The 10 Best and Worst Foods ... 26
Commandment IV - Double Your Fiber; Divide the Fat ... 28
Super Substitutes ... 41
Commandment V - Lots and Lots of Calcium and Iron ... 46
Commandment VI - Eat Your Fruits and Veggies ... 51
Commandment VII - Water, That Magic Potion ... 55
Commandment VIII - All About Salt and Sugar ... 57
Commandment IX - All About Alcohol, Caffeine, ... 64
                 Drugs, Artificial Sweeteners ... 64
Commandment X - Fad Diet Facts ... 69

The Healthy Meal Plan for Pregnancy ... 73
Your Grocery List for Health ... 75
The "What Abouts" of Pregnancy ... 78
  Morning Sickness ... 79
  Morning Sickness Prevention Plan ... 82
  Prenatal Multivitamin Mineral Supplements ... 84
  Smoking During Pregnancy ... 86
  Cravings ... 88
  Constipation ... 90
  Hemorrhoids ... 91
  Heartburn ... 92
  Exercise ... 94
  Swelling ... 97
  Toxemia ... 99
  Sleep ... 101
  Vegetarians ... 103
  Teenage Moms ... 104

multiple Births 106

What about Breastfeeding 109

What to Take to the Hospital 112

Pre-pregnancy Nutrition 113

How Does Your Baby Grow? 115

A Guide to Eating Out All over America 121

Nine Perfect Breakfast Menus with Recipes 135

Eight Easy Lunches with recipes 140

Nine Delicious Dinner Menus with Recipes 144

Quick Meals for the Fast Laners 160

Holiday and Party Entertaining for the Gourmet 163

A baby is God's opinion that
the world should go on.

Dear Mother to be,

New life has been created inside of you and you have been given a special privilege, the joy of nurturing your baby until birth! Eating well is a way to express your love for your baby right from the very start. Good nutrition is a gift that only _you_ can give your baby, but that gift goes on and keeps on giving! The food you eat is the food that makes your baby healthy, happy and well nourished. Such a blessed baby starts life with an advantage that carries on throughout a bright future; every aspect of your baby's life will be affected by nutrition that starts long before birth.

Yes, it takes a conscious effort to provide your baby with the very best. No maternal instinct draws you to a good diet and keeps you from what is harmful, but the reward of a healthy baby and child is worth the effort!

1

Once you begin to eat well, you will begin to feel well. You will have the advantage of the gift also because you will soon see a big difference in your energy level, your stamina, your skin, hair, nails and eyes right away. Beauty is an inside-out job. I have included my "Have it Your Way" mealplan to guide you to becoming perfectly "pregnant"!

Pamela Smith, R.D.

P.S. If you are not pregnant now but hope to be soon, be sure to see the special section for you, "Before the pregnancy is underway - Prepregnancy nutrition tips."

The 10 Commandments for Healthy Eating

I   Thou shalt never skip breakfast.

II Thou shalt eat every 2½ to 3 hours and have your healthy snack handy.

III Thou shalt never eat a protein without a carbohydrate.

IV Thou shalt double your fiber and halve your fat.

V   Thou shalt have lots and lots and lots of high-calcium and high iron foods.

3

VI Thou shalt believe your mother was right when she told you to eat your fruits and veggies.

VII Thou shalt drink at least 8 glasses of water each day.

VIII Thou shalt use a minimum of salt and sugar.

IX Thou shalt avoid alcohol, caffeine and artificial sweeteners.

X Thou shalt never go on a diet while pregnant, especially a fad diet.

4

1st Commandment: Thou shalt never skip breakfast.

If you want to start your day with a boundless energy level, your metabolism in high gear and proteins actively building you and your baby's new cells, then, "Thou shalt never skip breakfast."!

Think of your body as a campfire that dies down during the night and in the morning needs to be "stoked up" with wood to begin to burn vigorously again. Without stoking, the fire will die down with no flames or sparks. Your body is very similar; it awakens in a slowed, fasting state. You must "break the fast" with breakfast to rev up the body into high gear. If you choose not to eat breakfast, the body not only stays slowed down, but as is the case of the campfire, the metabolism will die down even more. Starving your body all day will have it dragging through the day in a slowed down metabolic state, unable to work efficiently for you and your When the evening "gorge" begins, much of the food will be wasted or stored as fat. All that food can't possibly be used up because the body isn't burning energy at a fast rate as the fire has already gone out. The food that comes in is like dumping an armful of fire-wood on a dead fire! Don't think for a minute that you are cutting calories by skipping breakfast or your healthy snacks; those calories would be burned by the higher metabolic rate. You are only starving your body and your baby of valuable carbohydrates that burn to give you energy and proteins that build your sweet baby.

Love doesn't make the world go around but it's what makes the ride worthwhile.

Breakfast is a vital tool for preventing nausea for it gives the blood sugars a needed boost and begins to neutralize stomach acidity. Don't ever make the mistake of skipping breakfast because you are queasy, it will make it worse! If you are fighting morning sickness, be sure to use the mealplan on page 82 that is especially designed to help you.

I bet you've said this, "If I skip breakfast, I don't really get hungry till much later in the day, but if I eat breakfast, I find myself hungry every few hours." You're right! This simply means your body is working correctly. When you starve your body in the morning, waste products are released into your system that temporarily depress your appetite and allow you to starve without feeling hungry for many hours. Unfortunately, these unhealthy products cross the placenta to the baby and you are 1- letting your body go into a slowed metabolic state, and 2- setting yourself up for a gorge, for as soon as you begin to eat, your appetite is really turned on! Not only will you overeat because your bloodsugar level has fallen so low, but like the campfire, your body will not be able to burn those calories well. Remember, your body just cannot handle such a large intake of food at one time; both you and your baby's needs go on 24 hours a day.

<u>Healthy Goal</u>: Start your day with a boundless energy level, your metabolism in high gear and proteins actively building that precious baby. <u>Never</u> skip breakfast!

The 7 Health Habits to Help You Live Longer

1. Buckle up - every time
2. Eat 3 meals a day plus healthy snacks.
3. Eat moderately. Don't overeat or undereat.
4. No cigarette smoking at all.
5. Exercise regularly - at least 20 minutes, 3 times a week.
6. Moderate to no use of alcohol
7. Get 7 to 8 hours of sleep a night.

Good health has more to do with everyday behavior and habits than with miracles of medical science.

Prevention of disease is far superior to cure!

9

2nd Commandment: Thou shalt eat every 2½ to 3 hours and have your healthy snack handy.

Smaller, more frequent meals will result in more energy, better nutrition for your baby's development and a healthy, proper weight gain.

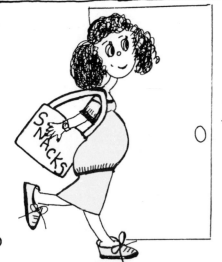

PARENT IN TRAINING CLASS

Remember the campfire story. Healthy snacking is very much like throwing wood on a fire all through the day to keep it burning well. You must keep your body fed the right thing at the right time to prevent nausea and fatigue. Also, understand that your appetite is almost totally controlled by your blood sugar. Keeping it even will help you prevent eating too much. You need to provide a constant source of nutrients in your bloodstream to be carried to the placenta. Not eating evenly through out the day endangers this flow and can leave you weak or dizzy.

Try to eat consistently and evenly each day including 3 meals with at least 2 healthy snacks. Ideally, you should eat 25% of your calories at breakfast, 25% at lunch, 25% at dinner and the other 25% in healthy snacks.

When most people think of snacks, they picture potato chips, candy, sodas. These types of snacks are "empty calories"; they provide high amounts of fat, sugar, salt, and calories but little or no vitamins or minerals.

11

A healthy snack is one that will provide you with needed nutrition and keep your blood sugar level from dropping too low, leaving you sleepy and craving sweets. It will keep your metabolism burning high, you and your baby's needs satisfied and still not load you with unwanted, unneeded fat, salt, sugar and calories.

Healthy Goal: If you want to take in food in the healthiest and most usable way, "Thou Shalt Eat A Healthy Meal or Snack Every 2½ to 3 Hours." The secret is to have your healthy snack handy — at home, in your car, in your desk drawer. You must plan ahead. When you go too long without food, you're likely to grab an unhealthy snack if you're not prepared.

Power Snack Ideas

- Whole grain crackers (5) and 2 oz. lowfat cheese
- Fresh fruit and 2 oz. lowfat cheese
- Nonfat yogurt (1 cup) blended with ½ cup unsweetened fruit. Try crushed pineapple, applesauce or the "All Fruit Preserves".
- Whole grain cereal (¾ cup) with 1 cup skim milk
- Popcorn (3 cups) sprinkled with 3 Tbsp. parmesan cheese
- Pita bread ½ with 2 oz. lowfat cheese, heated together. Add tomato sauce for pita pizza.
- Whole wheat English muffin with "Fat Free" cream cheese
- Warmed tortilla with 2 oz. lowfat cheese and salsa
- Noncreamed (1 cup) soup with celery sticks stuffed with "Fat Free" cream cheese.
- Homemade bran muffin with 8 oz. skim milk
- Rice cakes (2) with 1 Tbsp. natural peanut butter and 8 oz. skim milk.

More Power Snack Ideas

🍎 Sandwich (½). Great to freeze and take along
   to thaw.
🍎 Hardboiled egg with 3 whole wheat crackers
   and 8 oz. tomato juice
🍎 Small pop-top can of tuna, or chicken, packed
   in water with 5 whole wheat crackers
🍎 Trail mix (1 cup dry roasted, unsalted peanuts,
   1 cup dry roasted or raw sunflower seeds,
   2 cups raisins). Make in abundance and
   bag into ½ cup batches.
🍎 Yogurt dip ½ cup (see page 165 and 166) with
   raw veggies and 5 whole wheat crackers
🍎 Milk shake - skim milk (8 oz.) blended with
   ½ cup frozen fruit and 1 tsp. vanilla

14

<u>3rd Commandment: Thou shalt never eat a protein without a carbohydrate.</u>

Carbohydrate is 100% pure energy! It should be eaten with a protein to protect protein from being wasted as a less efficient source of energy. This allows protein to be used for its most important functions: building new cells, in you and in your baby, boosting your metabolism, building body muscle as well as providing for growth of the placenta and uterus, keeping body fluids in balance, healing and fighting infection, and making beautiful skin, hair and nails. Always remember, <u>carbohydrates burn</u> and <u>proteins build!</u>

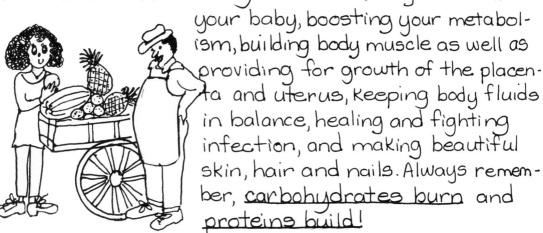

What is a carbohydrate and what does it do for me and my baby?

1- Anything that comes from a plant is a carbohydrate. The plant converts sunlight into carbohydrate then our bodies convert carbohydrates into energy! Carbohydrates are 100% pure energy!

2- Carbohydrates, and the vitamins and minerals they contain, are essential to your baby's growth and development.

3- Whole grain carbohydrates have not had the outer layers of grain removed so they contain many more vitamins, minerals and fiber than the refined, white (even though they're enriched,) products. Whole grain carbohydrates are rich in the B vitamins which are particularly crucial for the growth of your baby's cells, organ and limb formation, efficient digestion and metabolism of foods in you, and the prevention of anemia and possibly toxemia. Read more about anemia and toxemia on pages 49 + 99. Vitamin B·6, found in whole grain carbohydrates, is especially crucial in pregnancy. It is thought to be a major deterrent to nausea and fatigue in pregnancy, and appears to play a role in the prevention of toxemia.

4. You need at least 6 servings of whole grain carbohydrates each day. Always balance them with lots of low fat protein.

Let us not just live and let live, but live and help live.

Love gives and forgives.

Good things come in small packages?

17

Where are whole grain carbohydrates found?

100% whole wheat bread, crackers and pasta
   one serving = 1 slice bread, 5 crackers, ½ cup
   cooked pasta, 2 rice cakes or 2 Wasa Crispbreads.
Brown and wild rice - 1 serving = ½ cup cooked
Whole grain cereals such as Kellogg's Nutri-Grain,
   Shredded Wheat, Oatmeal, Wheatena - 3/4 cup
Corn or flour tortillas - 1 6 inch
Whole grain biscuits, muffins, rolls - 1
Popcorn, popped - 3 cups

   It is important to choose whole grain foods
at home to fill the void of what is missing in
restaurants. White, refined products still give
you carbohydrates for energy and some
vitamins but they are not the best for you
and your baby if eaten 100% of the time.

18

What is a protein and what does it do for me and my sweet baby?

1-Anything that comes from an animal gives you complete protein. A complete protein is one that supplies all the amino acids that are essential, those the body can't make or store. Legumes (dried beans and peanuts) although a plant food and incomplete in essential amino acids, are also excellent proteins.

2-The developing brain cells of your baby depend on your protein intake, as does the growth of the uterus and placenta. <u>Your need for protein increases greatly during pregnancy.</u> Your baby's development, both physically and intellectually, greatly depends on your protein intake!

19

3- Protein is the new you! Protein makes muscles that shape your body; it makes new hair, new nails and beautiful skin. It works to replace worn-out cells and to regulate your body's functions including fluid balance. During pregnancy, excessive swelling and fluid retention is most often caused by inadequate protein.

4- The amount of protein eaten is not the only secret to a healthy pregnancy. Protein is not stored, so it must be replenished frequently throughout the day, each and every day of your pregnancy. Remember, the protein and carbo- hydrates you eat are the fuels on which your body runs and your baby grows.

Misconceptions about Proteins

Never, never believe anybody or anything that tells you that you don't need protein, or to eat it only once a day. You are robbing your body of protein's healing and building power all day long.

The diets of our time have promised it to be the food to eat for weight loss and the truth is that an all-protein, no carbohydrate diet so imbalances the body that you do lose weight but all water and muscle, and little fat. Remember this after delivery as you begin to eat in such a way to return to your ideal weight. A balanced intake of protein with carbohydrate is essential to lose the right kind of weight while keeping your health.

21

Where are proteins found?

Complete protein is found in dairy products, eggs, fish, seafood, poultry, beef, pork and lamb.

One of the drawbacks of the American problem of overeating protein is that most of the popular protein foods are high in fat and fat is the major dietary risk factor in the killer diseases. By choosing the lower fat versions of protein foods you will get all of their goodness (protein, calcium, magnesium, iron and zinc) without the risk.

Ideal low fat protein sources

- Lowfat cheeses: Farmer's cheese, Mozzarella (part-skim) Weight Watcher's Natural cheddar, Kraft Natural Light, any part-skim milk cheese (1 oz. gives 1 oz. protein.)
- 1% or 2% lowfat cottage cheese - ¼ cup = 1 oz. protein
- Part-skimmed Ricotta - ¼ cup = 1 oz. protein
- Non-fat or Low-fat Yogurt - ½ cup = 1 oz. protein
- Lowfat and skimmed milk - skimmed milk is the only complete protein without fat. **8 ounces = 1 oz. protein**

22

🍎 Eggs - 1 egg = 1 oz. protein
🍎 Fish - 1 oz = 1 oz. protein
   ¼ cup water packed tuna or salmon = 1 oz. protein
🍎 Seafood - 5 shrimp, oysters, scallops or clams = 1 oz.
   ¼ cup crab or lobster = 1 oz. protein.
🍎 Chicken - 1 oz. = 1 oz. protein: 1 small split breast = 2 oz.
   1 large split breast = 3 oz., 1 leg = 1 oz., 1 leg-thigh combo
   = 3 oz and 1 small whole breast generally equals 4 oz.
🍎 Turkey - 1 oz. = 1 oz. protein
🍎 Veal - 1 oz. = 1 oz. protein
🍎 Lean Beef - 1 oz. = 1 oz. protein. Beef generally loses 25%
       in cooking
🍎 Lean, well trimmed pork 1 oz. = 1 oz. protein
🍎 Lean lamb 1 oz. = 1 oz. protein

   <u>Very Important!</u> While pregnant, your snack should include at least 2 oz. of protein and your meals should provide 3 to 4 ounces after cooking.

   If possible, please get a food scale and weigh your protein to <u>be sure</u> you are getting enough. Getting enough protein at the right time is what makes a healthy Mom and baby.

Where are incomplete proteins found?

Legumes: Soybeans, Pinto beans, Split peas, Lentils Kidney Beans, Black Beans, Red Beans, Navy Beans, Peanuts, Natural Peanut Butter

Legumes, although a plant food, contain enough valuable protein to be considered an excellent source of high-fiber, low-fat protein. They are considered "incomplete" proteins because they each lack sufficient amounts of one or more of the essential amino acids. They <u>must</u> be eaten with a grain (corn, wheat, rice oats) or a seed (sunflower, sesame) to be complete. Examples: peanut butter on bread, black beans over rice, beans and cornbread or tortillas, peanut and sunflower seed mix. Generally, 1/2 cup of cooked beans serves as 2 oz. of protein when mixed with an appropiate grain or seed and 3/4 cup will equal 3 oz. protein.

<u>Your Healthy Goal:</u> Eat 2 to 3 ounces of protein balanced with carbohydrates every 2 1/2 to 3 hours.

Beautiful Foods for Beautiful Bodies and Babies

There are certain foods that carry a powerful punch! They're loaded with the vitamins and minerals you and your sweet baby need to be healthy.

Get more of these into your diet and you'll see a big difference in your energy, stamina, hair, skin, nails and your general well being right away. Looking good and feeling good come from the inside.

<u>Healthy Goal</u>: Learn the 10 Best and 10 Worst Foods and increase the best and decrease or eliminate the worst and see how much better you feel and look!

25

The Ten Best Foods

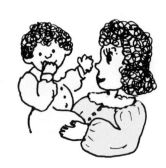

1 Broccoli

2 Chicken or turkey

3 Fish

4 Legumes (dried beans and peanuts)

5 Oranges

6 Potatoes - white and sweet

7 Skim or low-fat dairy products

8 Spinach

9 Strawberries

10 Whole grains - breads, cereals, crackers, rice, pasta

Ten Worst Foods

1. Artificial fruit drinks - nothing more than sugar, water with artificial flavor and coloring added.
2. Bacon, corned beef, ham, pastrami, salami and sausage Loaded with saturated fats, salt and preservatives
3. Breakfast or granola bars - candy bars rolled in oats! Loaded with sugar and fat.
4. Chocolate - high in saturated fat, caffeine and sugar.
5. Donuts - white flour and sugar fried in animal fat.
6. Hot dogs, bologna and all processed meats - high in saturated fat, salt and preservatives that have been linked to cancer.
7. Liver - high in iron as it may be, it is an animal's filter that collects the insecticides, poisons and cholesterol.
8. Snack chips and french fries - Triple threats: high in saturated fats, salt and calories.
9. Sodas - most have 12 teaspoons sugar per can.
10. Sugar

4th Commandment: Thou shalt double your fiber and halve your fat.

Grandma used to say "Eat your roughage" and now, years later, the Surgeon General says "Double your fiber."

Fiber is linked to the prevention of our killer diseases; heart disease, obesity, cancer and diabetes. The time has surely come to start increasing its amount in the diet. This can be done rather easily, not with "Fiber Pills" but by increasing your intake of whole grain breads and cereals, unprocessed bran, beans, fresh fruits and vegetables. These foods not only provide fiber but many other essential nutrients that cannot be obtained from other sources.

What is fiber?

1- Fiber is the part of plants not digested by the body.

2- There are 2 types of fiber: The water soluble fibers.

These are found in oats, barley, apples, dried beans and nuts and have been found to lower serum

28

cholesterol and triglyceride levels and to help control blood sugar levels. The _water insoluble fibers_ are found in wheat bran, whole grains and fresh vegetables and are excellent means of controlling chronic problems of pregnancy, constipation and hemorrhoids.

3. Think of fiber as a sponge which absorbs excess water in the GI tract to curtail diarrhea but provides a bulky mass which will pass more quickly and easily to relieve constipation, diverticulosis and possibly prevent hemorrhoids. Fiber needs water to make it work the way it should; ideally 8 to 10 glasses a day. The best way to drink water is to have a glass before and after every meal and snack rather than with a meal when it dilutes digestive functions. Try filling a 2 quart container with water each morning and make sure you have drunk it all before bedtime.

What does fiber do for me?

🍎 Fiber increases in the diet have been found to lower blood pressures as much as 10% with no other dietary changes.

🍎 Those population groups with high fiber intakes have a low incidence of many different types of cancers, particularly colon cancer.

🍎 Fiber's bulky mass in the intestine promotes fullness. This, combined with the fact that high fiber foods take longer to eat and stay in the stomach longer, keep you full longer.

🍎 Fiber serves as a "time-release capsule", slowly and evenly releasing sugars from digested carbohydrates into the bloodstream. This helps keep your energy levels even.

🍎 Fiber helps to protect against heart disease by lowering your level of "bad" LDL cholesteral.

30 🍎 Fiber regulates your G.I tract.

How do I double my fiber?

1. Use whole grains, such as brown rice, oats and WHOLE wheat rather than the white refined types. When purchasing, look for words such as 100% whole wheat with the word "whole" first in the ingredient list. Many manufacturers call products whole grain even if they contain only minimal amounts of **bran**. Brown dye does wonders in making food <u>look</u> healthy.
2. Eat vegetables and fruits with well washed skins on. You do need to peel the ones with wax on them.
3. Choose more raw and lightly cooked vegetables but in as non-processed form as possible. As a food becomes processed, ground, mashed, pureed or juiced, the fiber effectiveness is decreased.
4. Add a variety of legumes (dried beans and peanuts) to your diet.
5. It is important to choose whole grain foods at home to fill the void of what is missing in restaurants.

6. Add unprocessed raw bran to your cereals. Raw oat bran (from oatmeal) is particularly useful in reducing cholesterol levels; raw wheat bran is useful for a healthy, regular G.I. tract. Be careful to add bran gradually; begin with 1 teaspoon wheat bran and 1 teaspoon oat bran and slowly increase as your body adjusts to more fiber. Both types of bran may be purchased from your grocery store.

<u>Healthy goal</u>: Increase your fiber to keep your G.I tract regular; to help fight killer disease, to keep feeling full longer and to help you to say "no" to overeating by keeping your blood sugar level even.

Good health is everyone's major source of wealth. Without it, happiness is very difficult.

High Fiber Foods

Peanuts and peanut butter
Cooked dried beans
Sunflower and sesame seeds
Apples, Apricots, Peaches, Pears,
Bananas, Pineapple, Plums and Prunes.
Broccoli, Carrots, Corn, Lettuce, Peas,
Potatoes, including skins, Spinach
Bran, unprocessed wheat and oat
Bread, whole wheat
Brown rice
Cereals: whole grain, bran type,
Oatmeal, wheatena, whole wheat pasta

Don't be afraid to ask
dumb questions,
They're easier to handle
than dumb mistakes.

33

Refinement and Enrichment. A robbery that's legal.

Consider this story... A man was walking down the street when he was approached by a robber. The thief forced the man at gunpoint to take off all he was wearing - everything! After the man stripped, the thief said "I have just refined you." He then proceeded to return only four things; his watch, one shoe, his undershirt and necktie. The thief now proclaimed "I have just enriched you." Returning four nutrients and leaving out twenty one is what this enrichment thing is all about. A whole wheat berry contains approximately forty nutrients. When it is refined, every nutrient is affected and twenty one are completely lost. In the enrichment process, only four are added back. Don't be fooled by advertisements. White, even though it's enriched, is never nutritionally as good as whole grain.

34

All about fat: On your body and on your plate.

Fat is an essential nutrient needed in very limited amounts for lubrication of your body, for transporting fat-soluble vitamins and for fullness after eating. It is also a very concentrated way of getting calories and disease. Pregnancy does not give you the freedom to eat high-fat foods. Even though you may feel huge, there is a big difference between being fat and being pregnant! The healthy foods you eat are making you and your baby healthy; the excess fat you eat can make you fat and breeds more work after delivery.

Vital Facts about Fat

- Excess fat in the diet contributes to morning sickness and heartburn in pregnancy.
- Excess fat increases your risk of cancer, particularly breast, and colon cancer.

35

🍎 Excess fat intake increases your cholesterol and your risk of heart disease and stroke.

🍎 Excess fat, particularly saturated fat, has been shown to elevate blood pressure, regardless of the person's weight.

🍎 Excess fat increases your risk of gallblader disease.

🍎 Excess fat fed to animals with a genetic suscepti- bility to diabetes made them far more likely to develop the disease. People with a family history of diabetes should consider cutting their fat intake as one step in prevention of this disease in their own life.

🍎 Excess fat intake helps make you fat! One ounce of fat supplies twice the number of calories as an ounce of carbohydrate or protein. It's not the bread and potatoes that give you those excess calories; it's the butter and cream sauces.

<u>Healthy Goal</u>: As a general rule, the thing that makes you fat is fat. But do not confuse being pregnant with being fat.

Rating the Fats
Meats, Fish, Poultry and Legumes

High Fat (8 or more grams per servings)	Medium Fat (4 to 7 grams per serving)	Low Fat (3 or fewer grams per serving)
bacon	beef (rib roast, steak)	chicken
commercial peanut-butter	eggs	clams
corned beef	ham	crab
duck	lamb chops	fish
frankfurters	pork chops	lean beef (flank, round)
goose	liver	legumes
ground meat	veal cutlet	oysters
luncheon meats		scallops
pepperoni		shrimp
sausage		tuna (water packed)
spareribs		
tuna, (oil packed)		

37

Rating the Fats
Dairy Foods

High Fat (8 or more grams per servings)	Medium Fat (4 to 7 grams per serving)	Low Fat (3 or fewer grams per serving)
Cheese: American blue Brie Camembert cheddar brick Swiss Cream-whipping half-and-half commercial sour whole milk whole milk yogurt	Cheese: farmer's feta mozzarella Light Philadelphia part-skim cheddar part-skim ricotta string cheese creamed cottage 2% milk	Cheese: low fat- cottage cheese Laughing Cow non-fat cheese non-fat ricotta 1% or skim milk non-fat plain yogurt

38

Rating the Fats
Sauces and Toppings

High Fat (8 or more grams per servings)	Medium Fat (4 to 7 grams per serving)	Low Fat (3 or fewer grams per serving)
avocado butter coconut mayonnaise margarine olives oils shortening nuts: almonds pecans cashews walnuts	salad dressings nuts: Brazil peanuts	light sour cream light mayonnaise no-oil salad dressing

Rating the Fats
Soups

High Fat (8 or more grams per servings)	Medium Fat (4 to 7 grams per serving)	Low Fat (3 or fewer grams per serving)
all creamed soups all chunky soups pea with ham	beef noodle black bean chicken noodle chicken vegetable	low-sodium chicken bouillon lentil vegetable vegetable bean gazpacho onion

Note: In commercial soups, even low-fat ones, notice the sodium content, as it is probably high.

☼ Super Substitutes ☼

Small steps that can make a big, fat difference!

☼ Use skim milk, non-fat plain yogurt, skim milk cheese, low fat cottage cheese and "light" cream cheese instead of higher fat dairy products.

☼ Cream soups are the most common ingredient in any casserole and the worst nutritionally. They can easily be replaced with chicken stock, wine or a combination, thickened with cornstarch or arrowroot. Add your own fresh mushrooms for a healthy cream of mushroom base that so many recipes call for. For an even richer base, combine non-fat dry milk with chicken stock and thicken with cornstarch or arrowroot.

☼ Cold skim evaporated milk with a touch of honey and vanilla is a super whipped topping. It does take longer to whip but the nutritional gains are worth it. You can also use 2 cups skim milk with one teaspoon lemon juice, chill well, then whip. Never use non-dairy whipped toppings. They are chemical non foods, loaded with saturated fat and sugar.

41

More Super Substitutes

♡ Basting with butter is another frustrating recipe direction for a healthy gourmet. Adapt instead by basting with tomato, lemon juice or stock.

♡ Use only _natural_ peanut butter. Avoid commercial peanut butter! Commercial peanut butter is not much more than shortening and sugar but fresh ground peanut butter is a great source of protein. If you have trouble switching from the commercial type, begin by mixing it half and half with natural. Gradually increase the portion of natural.

♡ Try using legumes (dried beans and peas) as a main dish or a meat substitute for a high nutrition, low fat meal.

♡ Use canola or olive oil for salads or cooking. They are valuable sources of monounsaturated fat, but they are still fat so use sparingly.

42

More Super Substitutes

- ♡ Purchase tuna packed in water rather than oil.
- ♡ Use non-stick sprays because they enable you to brown meats without grease.
- ♡ Dilute soy sauce or tamari sauce half and half with water and add 1 teaspoon lemon juice. It increases the flavor and reduces the salt. You may also use low sodium soy sauce.
- ♡ If using canned or frozen fruits, use only unsweetened, without sugar, packed in its own juices.
- ♡ Use more vanilla and spices in recipes. This will enable you to cut down more on the sugar since vanilla and spices enhance the impression of sweetness and flavor and have almost no calories.
- ♡ Healthy bread crumbs can be made by processing toasted, whole wheat bread in a food processor or blender.

43

More Super Substitutes

🍎 Use whole grains anytime a recipe calls for white. Use brown rice or whole wheat pasta instead of white; whole grain crackers instead of saltines, etc.

🍎 Substitute fiber and water for laxatives. A laxative isn't the healthy way to get rid of anything; fiber and water are!

🍎 Use two egg whites in place of one whole egg. Egg whites are pure protein and egg yolks are pure fat. You may want to try some of the egg substitutes on the market now.

🍎 Great potato toppings: salsa, nonfat sour cream, plain nonfat yogurt, blended till smooth nonfat cottage cheese, chives, grated parmesan.

Which is the lesser of two evils; food going to waste or to your waist?

For the flavor of butter, but the polyunsaturated to saturated fat ratio and spreadability of corn oil margarine (minus the yellow dyes and preservatives), mix up <u>Better Butter</u>

1 cup canola oil
1 cup (2 sticks) butter
Blend butter till fluffy, slowly pour in oil until well blended.

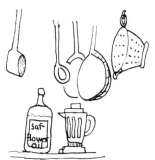

If you use margarine, the soft, squeeze kind is best, (less hydrogenation) then tub, then stick. Be sure it's 100% corn oil, safflower or canola oil.

5th Commandment: Thou shalt have lots and lots and lots and lots of high calcium and high iron foods.

What is calcium and why is it so important to me and my baby?

Calcium is a mineral needed by your body and baby's for the development of strong bones and teeth. It is particularly crucial in the last 3 months of pregnancy when the baby's bone formation is taking place at an accelerated rate. During this time the body's need doubles from 1000 to 2000 mg. Every hour of the day throughout your pregnancy, your baby draws calcium from your body's supply. Your baby <u>will</u> get calcium. If you do not eat adequate food sources to supply the need, the baby will draw from your reserves. The short range symptoms of an inadequate calcium intake during pregnancy may be sleeplessness, irritability, muscle cramps in the legs and uterine pain. The long range effect may be osteoporosis, a crippling disease of brittle bones.

You require calcium in your diet all of your life but particularly during your pregnancy! You need at least 1200 mg. of calcium each day, and, like protein, it will best be utilized if eaten in smaller, more evenly distributed amounts through the day. The required amount can be obtained in 4 servings of high calcium foods.

The task ahead of you is never as great as the power behind you. You have been born with a genetic heritage for wellness. Claim that power!

What are high calcium foods?

Milk, 1 cup is one serving = 250 mg.
Cheese - 1 1/2 oz
Yogurt - 1 cup (low fat)
Cottage Cheese - 1 1/2 cups
Salmon, water packed - 5 oz.
Collard or turnip greens
Broccoli - 2 cups
Dried beans, cooked - 2 1/2 cups
Tofu or fortified soy milk - 1 cup
Part-skimmed Ricotta - 1/2 cup

Like magic, babies touch the world with love.

What is anemia and why do you need high iron foods to prevent it ?

Along with increased protein and calcium needs, a pregnant woman must be careful to eat enough foods high in iron. During the last trimester of pregnancy, your baby will store enough iron for the first few months of life. If you do not take in enough iron each day, your baby will draw from your reserves. Consequently, iron-deficiency anemia is all too easy to fall into. A woman with anemia tires easily and is very susceptible to infections. Her baby has a greater chance of being anemic during the first year of life. The eating guidelines we have discussed so far, small amounts of protein and whole grains eaten evenly during the day, will help you absorb iron most efficiently. Foods high in vitamin C also help you absorb it. Eating citrus foods or juices as well as vegetables such as those in the cabbage family (broccoli, cauliflower, Brussels sprouts and cabbage) along with high iron foods, will enhance their already important role.

Tea, coffee, colas and chocolate hinder the absorption of iron due to their tannic or oxalic acid content so never drink them with a meal. Water is the best beverage!

Be sure you choose plenty of high iron foods such as dried fruits, well cooked oysters and clams, dried beans and peas, whole grains, and if you are a meat eater, lean red meats and poultry. Your doctor may recommend supplemental iron to add to your intake from food. These are best absorbed when taken with your power snacks, between meals.

Citrus fruit, (not the juice if you are experiencing heartburn) enhances absorption. All vitamin C foods do. Like calcium and protein, iron is a mineral that the more you take in at one time, the less the body absorbs, so spread it out all day long.

<u>6th Commandment: Thou shalt believe</u>
<u>your mother was right when she told</u>
<u>you to eat your fruits and veggies.</u>

What are the "best" fruits and vegetables
for pregnancy?

<u>All</u> fruits and vegetables make up an
enormously important part of your healthy
diet. They provide a storehouse of vitamins
and minerals, they provide substances
that serve as protectors against
disease and they are valuable sources
of fiber and fluids - all in all - tasty,
healthy, low calorie munchies.
Your main supply of vitamin
A and Folic acid and all of
your vitamin C will come
from fruits and vegetables.
One serving is ½ cup cooked veggies
or fruit, ½ cup fruit or vegetable juice or 1 medium
fruit or vegetable. Choose 6 a day.

You may not be able to tell a book by its cover, but you can sure choose a vegetable by its color! Generally, the more vivid in color the fruit or vegetable is, the higher in essential nutrients for you and your baby. That deep orange-red coloring in carrots, sweet potatoes, cantaloupes, apricots, and strawberries is a sign of its vitamin A content.

Dark green leafy vegetables like greens, spinach, romaine lettuce, broccoli and Brussels sprouts are also loaded with vitamin A but have an extra bonus of being the source of Folic acid, a "must have" in pregnancy. To meet your need of this valuable nutrient, have 2 servings of fresh or cooked tender-crisp dark, green leafys each day. Vitamin C is found in more than just citrus, it is also power-packed into strawberries, cantaloupe, tomatoes, green peppers, broccoli and those little Brussels sprouts. Remember, if they're loaded with color, they're loaded with nutrition.

Tips to retain those valuable vitamins and minerals:

♡ Buy vegetables that are as fresh as possible, and when not possible, frozen is the next best choice. (Avoid those frozen with butter or sauces.)

♡ Use peelings and outer leaves of vegetables whenever possible because that's where the highest concentration of nutrients is found. Peeling is a waste of time and nutrients 53

- Store vegetables in airtight containers in the refrigerator.
- Do not store vegetables in water. Too many vitamins are lost.
- Do not boil. Steam or microwave in a minimum of water.
- Cook vegetables until tender crisp, not mushy. Overcooked vegetables lose their flavor along with their vitamins.

We are not born as the partridge in the woods, or the ostrich in the desert, to be scattered everywhere; but we are to be grouped together and brooded by love and reared day by day in that first of all churches, the family.

Henry Ward Beecher

7th Commandment: Thou shalt drink at least 8 glasses of water a day.

Because water makes up 92% of our blood plasma, 80% of our muscle mass, 60% of our red blood cells and 50% of everything else in our body, it is vitally important for health, especially in pregnancy! Water is as essential a nutrient as the other 5: carbohydrates, proteins, fats, vitamins and minerals.

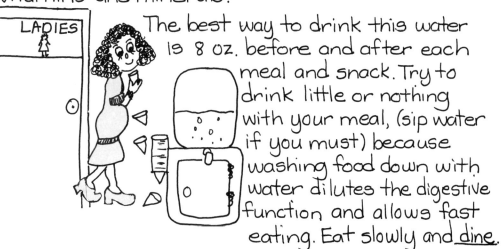

The best way to drink this water is 8 oz. before and after each meal and snack. Try to drink little or nothing with your meal, (sip water if you must) because washing food down with water dilutes the digestive function and allows fast eating. Eat slowly and dine.

LADIES

55

Remember: Do not rely on your thirst mechanism. It will replace 35 to 40% of your needs. Also, don't rely on your intake of other fluids. No other liquid works like water. If you do not take in adequate water, your body fluids will be thrown out of balance, you may experience fluid retention, con-stipation, unexplained weight gain and loss of that natural thirst mechanism.

<u>Healthy Goal</u>: Begin to focus on drinking wonderful, essential water and drink enough!

Try a glass of warm water and the juice of a lemon. It's a mild, natural diuretic and laxative. If you are drinking tap water, you may find the taste will improve with refrigeration for 24 hours (the chlorine dissipates). Water is particularly refreshing with fresh lemon or lime slices. You may find you enjoy bottled water, club soda or seltzer water as a nice treat.

8th Commandment: Thou shalt use a minimum of salt and sugar.

All of the commandments up to this point have focused on the nutrients vital to wellness. This one points to the need to avoid some things which do not benefit the body, but rather can cause harm if eaten to excess. The problem with salt and sugar is that they can easily cause a problem with overindulgence. If you are a person who may be taking in these to excess, if you have the "more you have, the more you want" syndrome, this commandment is for you!

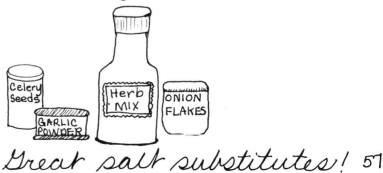

Great salt substitutes! 51

Salt - Don't Pass It!

"Please pass the salt" is a common phrase which is overused by most Americans. We need to shake the habit! The taste for salt is conditioned, and as you begin to use less of it, your taste will change so that you will enjoy foods more without it. Be patient with yourself and your family, but begin to gradually cut back on its use in cooking and cut out completely those snack foods that are triple threats: high in salt, fat and calories.

What is salt?

Its chemical name is sodium chloride... with sodium being the more important in terms of health. Everyone requires some sodium and although your need for sodium during pregnancy actually increases, there's more than enough sodium naturally present in foods to supply this requirement. Sodium should not be severely restricted during pregnancy but if you use salt to an extreme, it would be wise to begin to cut back on its overuse. Most of us consume 5 to 25 times more than we need.

Effects of salt.

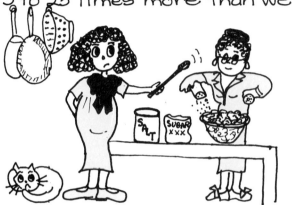

Excessive sodium is indicated in many diseases, especially hypertension, (high blood pressure) and kidney disease. Excess salt causes temporary buildup of body fluids in your system. This makes it diffucult for your heart to pump blood through the cardiovascular system, and the results may be high blood pressure or excessive swelling. Although some fluid retention is normal in pregnancy, if you begin to swell to an extreme, you will probably be asked to cut back on your use of high salt foods. Don't wait; begin to start changing how you eat now.

Where do I get sodium and how can I shake the habit?

1. Cutting back on your use of more highly processed foods and salty snacks will substantially reduce your sodium intake.

2. Leave the salt shaker off the table. You'll quickly begin to enjoy the natural flavor of your food without covering them with salt. Try substituting herbs and spices for some of the salt.

3. Attempt to cook with herb blends rather than salt to add new flavors to cooking. Try making your own and keep in a large holed shaker right by the stove where your salt used to be.
   Seasoning blends: (I) 2 tsp. dry mustard, 1 1/2 tsp. oregano, 1 tsp. marjoram, 1 tsp. thyme, 1 tsp. garlic powder, 1 tsp. curry powder, 1/2 tsp. onion powder, 1/2 tsp. celery seed. (II) 1 Tbs. garlic powder, 1 Tbs. dry mustard, 1 Tbs. paprika, 1 1/2 tsp. pepper, 1 tsp. basil, 1/2 tsp. thyme.

4- Watch out for these high sodium foods :
- Any food pickled or brine cured, like sauerkraut, pickles.
- Any food salt-cured or smoked, like ham and bacon.
- Salted snack foods like salted top crackers and chips.
- Condiments, like soy sauce and ketchup. Use in moderation.
- Convenience foods, like frozen dinners and instant soup mix.
- Most canned foods like canned soups, vegetable juices, canned vegetables. Check label for sodium content.

Cheer up! Sodium does not have to be cut out completely; you only need to be aware of its sources and begin to cut back on excess use. Accept the challenge of learning to cook and enjoy foods without the usual added fat and salt. Included are many wonderful recipes that are a great place to start.

Sugar: How sweet it isn't!

Sugar is called by many names - honey, brown sugar, corn syrup, fructose, etc, but it's all sugar! Occasional use of sugar is possible for some but impossible for others. Those that are very sensitive to blood sugar fluctuations will be hurt by "just a little bit" not by calories, but by the effect it has on their body. The "seesaw effect" that sugar has seems to result in a "more you have, more you want" addiction. A heavy sugar intake causes a quick rise in blood sugar that will be followed by a quick fall. That dip in blood sugar triggers "eating for a lift" to relieve fatigue. Usually the food is, again, high in sugar and the "seesaw effect" continues!

Sugar has been shown to cause dental cavities, obesity, and high triglycerides as well as wreaking havoc in the control of diabetes and hypoglycemia.

Sugary foods may be replacing other healthier foods (such as fruit) which would contribute vitamins, minerals and fiber.

62

Most high sugar snacks (candy bars, cookies, donuts, etc.) are also loaded with saturated fats and calories - another triple threat to good health.

<u>Healthy Goal</u>: Cut back on your daily use of sugar or sweets and eat fruit to satisfy your natural craving for sugar. Sugar is not worth robbing yourself of your precious energy and stamina.

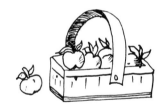

Anyone can count the seeds in an apple but only God can count the apples in a seed.

9th Commandment: Thou shalt avoid alcohol, caffeine, drugs and artificial sweeteners.

What about alcohol?

There is absolutely no safe amount of alcohol for you to drink during pregnancy. Studies have shown that babies born to mothers that drink have lower IQ's and higher rates of joint and heart defects. Even babies that are born to mothers that drink in moderation may be affected negatively; studies have shown that frequent intake of even two alcoholic drinks a day increases the risk of delivering a baby with physical and developmental problems. For some women, even smaller amounts of alcohol may produce the same risks, and "binge" drinking appears to carry an even higher risk. Research has not given us a magical quantity of what is "safe" excepting <u>none</u>. If you choose to drink alcohol, even sparingly, talk it over with your doctor.

64 Remember: <u>When in doubt, leave it out!</u>

What about caffeine?

Caffeine is a stimulant that activates the central nervous system of you and your baby. It accelerates the body, causing agitation, increased heart rate and dilation of the blood vessels. A baby does not benefit from this kind of stimulation. Although there are no cases of birth defects attributed to caffeine intake, we do know caffeine crosses the placenta and has been found in fetal blood. An F.D.A study advises pregnant women to be prudent about their intake. Reduce your intake to below 150 mg. per day, (less than 2 cups of coffee, tea or soda) or better yet, give it up altogether. Remember, caffeine is in cocoa, colas, many sodas and even chocolate. When in doubt, leave it out!

What about drugs?

Drugs you take can cross the placenta and damage your developing baby. Never use a drug of any kind unless your doctor has prescribed or approved it. Remember that even simple aspirin can interfere with your baby's blood supply and lengthen your labor, so check with your doctor for an OK for even what seems to be insignificant medication. When in doubt, leave it out!

Maturity is the ability to live in peace with that which we cannot change.

It's good to let a little sunshine out as well as in.

What about artificial sweetners?

A major controversy comes into play as you start looking towards decreasing your intake of sugar; the question of artificial sweetners. There are no absolutes in the safety of chemicals - be it saccharin, aspartame or any new one to come. It will be years before we have all the answers. In the case of aspartame (marketed as Nutrasweet), in the short time since it has appeared on the market, cautions concerning its use have accelerated with questions concerning its allergic reaction in some; its dangger with possible breakdown in hot foods and its effect on children and the unborn. The battle will continue; for even though it is made from natural sources, it is still made in a laboratory and is not found in nature. There are endless possibilities

67

for problems to occur with its frequent use. As bad as sugar is and with all of the health hazards indicated in its overuse - at least it's not chemical and it's been used for centuries.

Also understand that as long as you continue to use sugar-laden foods or sugar substitutes, you will keep your taste buds alive for sugar. The goal is to begin to cut back on its use so that the need is not there for everything to taste sweet. Allow your taste buds to change so that the desire for sweetness can be met in a safer way, from fruits and other naturally sweet foods that are God's natural outlets for our inborn sweet preference. <u>When in doubt, leave it out !</u>

Nothing keeps a person's feet on the ground like having a little responsibility placed on their shoulders.

10th Commandment: Thou shalt never go on a diet during pregnancy, especially a fad diet.

How much should I eat?

You require more calories during pregnancy but only 15 to 20% more! You don't need to double your normal intake just because you're eating for two. It's quality, not quantity you are now seeking. Although you may need only 150 extra calories a day for the first 3 months and 400 extra each day the remaining months, your vitamin and mineral needs jump as much as 25% to 100%. These few extra calories don't really amount to that much food (you can get that many in a large piece of pie), so you must choose carefully what you eat to pack in the higher amounts of vitamins, minerals and protein you require.

69

There is no room for foods that are high in calories but low in nutrition ... since you must consider that sweet baby inside of you that you and you alone are nurturing.

What about weight gain ?

The weight gain controversy has been swinging back and forth like a pendulum for years. A major fallacy is the belief that the less weight gained during pregnancy, the better. This misconception, widely held a few decades ago, was based on the belief that women who gained little or no weight would be less likely to develop complications during pregnancy and would have smaller, more easily delivered babies. Research has proven both theories wrong, and we now know that a healthy weight increase is 25 to 30 pounds gained evenly throughout the pregnancy. The pattern of gaining weight is at least as important as the total amount; the goal should be a slow, steady gain. You should

gain 4-5 lbs. the first three months and approximately 3-4 lbs. each of the remaining 6 months.
The amount of weight gain appears to positively
affect your baby's health far beyond the birth
weight - maybe for the baby's entire life.
Remember that a healthy weight gain
is not just fat weight but is instead
specific body changes that weigh
more on the scale. About 7 ½ lbs. will
be baby; 4-5 lbs. come from an increase in the size of the breasts
and uterus; another 9 lbs. is con-
tributed by a combination of the
placenta, amniotic fluid, extra blood
volume and other fluids; and
another 6-7 lbs. will be reserved energy
stores. Never try to lose weight during
pregnancy - even if you are overweight. Restrict-
ing calories limits the chances of getting the
right amount of nutrients (such as calcium, iron,

and protein.) If you diet, your own body fat will be used for energy and will form ketones, a waste product. Ketones can cross the placenta and may damage your baby's brain cells. This is your first chance to directly impact your baby's health. You will have a lifetime to lose weight! Use this time as a chance to break the "Diet Mentality". Learn what good eating is all about so that it will be possible to lose weight effectively _after_ that precious baby is born, as a side effect of eating well! What a wonderful time it is now to start leaving out sugar-laden foods and salty, high fat snacks and start replacing them with delicious but healthy foods.

A human being is happiest and most successful when dedicated to a cause outside his own individual, selfish satisfaction. Benjamin Spock

A NUTRITION PLAN TO ENSURE A HEALTHY DAY FOR YOU AND YOUR BABY

<u>BREAKFAST</u>—(within 1/2 hour of arising)

SIMPLE CHO:	1 serving fresh fruit
COMPLEX CARBO:	2 slice whole wheat toast OR 1 English Muffin/bagel OR 2 homemade muffins OR 1-1/2 cups cereal (with added bran)
PROTEIN:	2 oz. lowfat cheese or 1/2 cup lowfat cottage cheese OR 2 eggs (only 2 times/wk) or 1/2 cup egg substitute OR 1-1/2 cups skim milk or nonfat yogurt for cereal

<u>MORNING SNACK</u>

CARBOHYDRATE:	1 fresh fruit AND 5 whole grain crackers OR 2 rice cakes or Wasa OR 1 slice whole wheat bread
PROTEIN:	2 oz. part-skim or fat free cheese OR lean meat OR 1 cup nonfat yogurt OR 1/2 cup lowfat cottage cheese

<u>LUNCH</u>

SIMPLE CHO:	1 serving fresh fruit
COMPLEX CARBO:	2 slices bread OR 1 baked potato OR 1 whole wheat pita
PROTEIN:	3-4 oz. (cooked poultry, fish, seafood, lean beef or lowfat cheese) OR 1 cup cooked legumes
HEALTHY MUNCHIES: (optional)	Raw vegetables as desired (up to 2 cups) with lemon juice, vinegar, mustard or no-oil salad dressing
ADDED FAT: (optional)	1 Tbsp. light mayonnaise OR 1 tsp. oil OR 1 Tbsp. salad dressing

<u>AFTERNOON SNACK</u>—Repeat earlier snack choices OR 1/2 cup Trail Mix (page 14)

<u>DINNER</u>

SIMPLE CHO:	1 fresh fruit AND 1 cup nonstarchy vegetables
COMPLEX CARBO:	1 cup rice or pasta OR 1 cup starchy vegetables
PROTEIN:	3 to 4 oz. cooked skinless poultry, seafood, fish, lean beef OR 1 cup cooked legumes
HEALTHY MUNCHIES: **(optional)**	Raw vegetables (up to 2 cups) as desired with lemon juice, vinegar, or no-oil salad dressing
ADDED FAT: **(optional)**	May use 1 tsp. olive or canola oil OR 1 Tbsp. salad dressing OR 1 tsp. butter or margarine

<u>NIGHT SNACK</u>—1 cup cereal with 1 cup skim milk or nonfat yogurt AND 1 serving fruit

74

GROCERY LIST
GRAINS

<u>100% Whole Wheat Bread</u> - look for "whole" as first word of ingredient list

<u>Whole Wheat Bagels, English Muffins, Hamburger Buns and Pita bread</u>

<u>Whole Wheat Pasta</u> (best variety at Natural Food Store)

<u>Whole Wheat Pastry Flour</u> (best for muffins, pancakes, etc.) at Natural Food Store

<u>Brown Rice, Instant Brown Rice, and Wild Rice</u>

<u>Whole Grain Crackers and Such</u>

    Crispbread - Wasa (2=1 Complex Carbo) and Kavli (4=1 Complex Carbo)

    Crispy Cakes (2=1 Complex Carbo)

    Guiltless Gourmet No Oil Tortilla Chips (1 oz. = 1 Complex Carbo)

    Harvest Crisp (5=1 Complex Carbo)

    Mini-Rice Cakes (4=1 Complex Carbo)

    Rice Cakes (2=1 Complex Carbo)

    Ry-Krisp (3=1 Complex Carbo)

<u>Great Cereals</u> (Generally, 3/4 cup = 1 Complex Carbo)

    Cheerios (General Mills)

    Grape-Nuts (concentrated; 1/4 cup=1 Complex Carbo)

    Muesli (Ralston)

    Nutrigrain Almond-Raisin or Wheat (Kellogg's)

    Puffed Rice, Puffed Wheat (Lightweight; 1 cup=1 Complex Carbo)

    Oatmeal, Oat Bran

    Raisin Squares (Kellogg's)

    Shredded Wheat, Shredded Wheat 'N Bran (Nabisco)

    Unprocessed Wheat Bran

    Wheatena

DAIRY AND DELI

Cheese (lowfat= less than 5 grams fat per ounce)

    Alpine Lace "Lean and Free"

    Cottage Cheese (Fat Free or 1%)

    Cream Cheese (Kraft "Light" Tub or Fat Free, Healthy Choice Fat Free)

    Farmer's

    Jarlsberg Lite

    Kraft Light Naturals

    Mozzarella (Nonfat, Part-skim or String Cheese)

    Parmesan (fresh grated)

    Ricotta (Nonfat or Part-skim)

    String Cheese - try MooTown Snackers Light

    The Laughing Cow Reduced Calorie (needs no refrigeration)

    Weight Watcher's Natural

Eggs or Egg Substitutes

Milk (Skim or 1% lowfat)

Margarine (Fleischmann's Squeeze is best) or Butter

Nonfat Plain Yogurt (may add all fruit jam to sweeten)

Stonyfield Farms Nonfat Yogurt (sweetened with fruit and fruit juice)

MISCELLANEOUS

<u>Assorted variety of seasonal fresh fruits and vegetables</u>;
DON'T FORGET: bananas, apples, oranges, melon, strawberries, romaine lettuce, broccoli, carrots, tomatoes, squash, white and sweet potatoes. Also buy raisins and canned, unsweetened applesauce, crushed pineapple.

<u>Mayonnaise</u> - May use a tsp. of traditional mayonnaise OR
1 Tbsp. Miracle Whip Lite OR Kraft Light and Lively OR Hellman's Light (Believe it or not, light mayo is healthier than fat free - it has less chemicals and sugar)

<u>Olive oil, Canola oil</u>

<u>Natural Peanut Butter</u>
May buy fresh ground at deli OR from health food store

<u>Popcorn</u> - Orville Redenbacher's Light Natural Microwave OR Pop Weaver Light

<u>Dry roasted, unsalted peanuts and shelled sunflower seeds</u>

<u>Low Calorie Salad Dressings</u>

May prefer to use 1 Tbsp. regular dressing with lemon juice OR vinegar
Bernstein's Low Calorie Cheese Italian OR Vinegarette; Pritikin; Kraft "No Oil" Dressing; Barendorf's

<u>No Sugar Jam</u> - try Sorrell Ridge, Polaner Preserves or Smuckers Simply Fruit (Fruit Only Preserves) OR Welch's Totally Fruit

77

breastfeeding? sleep? swelling? gas?
morning sickness? heartburn?
exercise? constipation?
smoking? multiple births?
teenage moms? cravings?
pre-pregnancy? hospital stay?
pregnant vegetarians? prenatal supplemen
hemorrhoids? toxemia?

The "What Abouts"
of Pregnancy

What about morning sickness?

During pregnancy, especially during the first 3 months, your hormones are fluctuating wildly and so is your blood sugar level. This can lead to fatigue, queaziness and nausea. Although the exact cause is unknown, we do know that an even, frequent intake of protein and carbohydrate all through the day will work to keep your blood sugar stable and help to <u>prevent sickness before it hits</u>! As you might have noticed, once you begin to feel bad, it's too late. You <u>can</u> prevent the blood sugar dips. <u>Eat when you are feeling your best. Start before you even get out of bed</u>, when your blood sugar is lowest.

CRACKERS

79

with some crackers kept at your bedside. If whole wheat is not appealing at this time, try a milder rice cracker. Relax in bed while eating them and continue to <u>lay still for 10 to 15 minutes.</u> Follow this with a small balanced breakfast after getting up, and continue to <u>eat small snacks every two hours all through the day and evening.</u> Your night snack is the beginning of a well morning. You will also sleep more restfully and wake more refreshed. Don't wait until you are hungry to eat! Eat your small meals and snacks to prevent getting hungry, to prevent your blood sugars from dropping, to prevent morning sickness.

Avoid fats in your food as much as possible as these stay in your stomach longer and are harder to digest. Avoid drinking liquids with meals, instead drink after the meal.

It will take your body 2 to 3 days to stabilize, and once you begin to feel better, continue to eat small meals for peak energy and wellness.

Healthy goal: Eat small meals every 2 to 3 hours to prevent sickness rather than eating to try to cure it. In the case of morning sickness, "An ounce of prevention really is worth a pound of cure!"

Follow the "no nausea" meal plan designed to prevent morning sickness.

A child is a person who can't understand why someone would give away a perfectly good kitten.

MEAL PLAN TO COMBAT MORNING SICKNESS...

It will take 2 to 3 days for your body to stabilize so don't give up!

BEFORE GETTING OUT OF BED: **5 whole grain crackers.** Relax for 10 to 15 minutes.

UPON RISING: 6 oz. unsweetened juice (no citrus)

BREAKFAST - within 1/2 hour of arising - 7:00 a.m.

COMPLEX
  CARBO: 1 slice of 100% whole wheat bread OR 1/2 whole wheat
             English Muffin OR 1 cup cereal WITH added bran*

PROTEIN: 1 oz. lowfat cheese OR 1 egg OR 6 oz. skim milk for cereal

SIMPLE
  CARBO: 1 piece of fresh fruit

1st AM SNACK — 9:00 a.m.

CARBO: 5 whole grain crackers OR 1 pc. fruit OR 2 rice cakes
PROTEIN: 1 oz. cheese/lean meat

2nd AM SNACK — 11:00 AM - 1/4 cup Trail Mix (see page 14)

LUNCH - 1:00 p.m.

COMPLEX
  CARBO: 2 slices of bread OR 1 baked potato OR 10 crackers
             OR 1 whole wheat pita

PROTEIN: 2 oz. cooked (poultry, fish, roast beef, lowfat cheese)

SIMPLE
  CARBO: 1 small piece of fresh fruit OR 1 cup non-creamed soup

HEALTHY
  MUNCHIE: Raw vegetable salad, if desired

ADDED
  FAT: 1 tsp. mayonnaise OR 1 Tbsp. dressing

1st AFTERNOON SNACK - **3:00 p.m.** Repeat earlier snack choices
OR 1/2 cup plain yogurt mixed with
1/2 cup fruit OR 1 Tbsp no sugar jam

2nd AFTERNOON SNACK — **5:00 p.m.** Repeat earlier snack choices

DINNER — **7:00 p.m.**

COMPLEX CARBO:	1 cup rice or pasta OR 1 cup starchy vegetable
PROTEIN:	2-3 oz. cooked (chicken, turkey, fish, seafood, lean roast beef, 1/2 cup beans)
SIMPLE CARBO:	1 cup non-starchy vegetable OR 1 pc. fresh fruit
HEALTHY MUNCHIE:	Raw vegetable salad, if desired
ADDED FAT:	May use 1 tsp. of margarine/butter or olive oil; OR 2 tbsp. sour cream OR 1 tbsp. salad dressing

NIGHT SNACK — any "Power Snack" (page 13) or 3/4 cup cereal with 1/2 cup skim milk

*Begin adding 1 tsp. bran, gradually increase to 2 Tbsp.

**"Better Butter" recipe on page 45

83

What about prenatal multivitamin mineral supplements?

If you follow the recommended nutritional guidelines and make healthy choices, the chances are that you will get the vitamins and minerals you need during pregnancy. Your doctor may have prescribed a prenatal multivitamin-mineral supplement for you to take. The supplement will fill in the needs you may have not met that day, but don't let your prenatal vitamin and mineral supplement give you the false sense of security that you don't have to be concerned about your diet. No supplement can come close to meeting your need for calcium. To sum it up, don't believe you can take a vitamin supplement to replace good food and don't believe poor eating can ever be solved by a pill.

Take as directed and be sure not to medicate

yourself with additional dietary supplements, and never take a supplement without your doctors advice. Pregnancy is no time to experiment! Many vitamins and minerals, if taken in additional megadose quantities, can seriously harm you and your unborn precious child. Your baby's liver, the organ that breaks down or stores extra vitamins, is still underdeveloped and needless nutrients may circulate for a long time causing tissue and organ damage. Consistently high doses of vitamin C could make your baby "dependent" on it; that is, requiring unusually high amounts of vitamin C after birth that can't be met through normal feeding.

<u>Healthy goal:</u> Take your prenatal supplement as prescribed but remember, just because a little is good, more is not necessarily better!

What about

Smoking in Pregnancy?

If there is ever a time you should give up smoking it is when you are pregnant! Smoking lowers the amount of oxygen that reaches your baby. It may also reduce the amount of nutrients available to the baby from the placenta. Studies show that there are 2½ times more premature births and 3 times more low-weight babies born to smoking mothers. Smoking has also been associated with increased risk of miscarriage, stillbirth, placental bleeding and possibly lower IQ's in children. And don't forget, if you stop smoking now, you will be providing a home for your baby to be born into that is free from smoke. Infants of smoking parents tend to come down with more respiratory illnesses. Be kind to that precious baby you and you alone are nurturing and make its home, both before and after its birth, a healthy place to be.

A Grandmother is someone who tells my mother and father if they're raising me wrong.

A Grandmother is a second mother or even better. She spoils you and says yes when your mother says no.

A Grandmother is nothing like a mother. She lets you put back your vegetables when your mother isn't looking.

87

What about cravings ?

Many people feel that pregnant women crave foods their bodies need. Actually, the opposite is true! Even intelligent, healthy women can develop a craving for bizzare substances such as laundry starch or clay. They should not be reluctant to discuss this problem with their physician, for it may be an indirect sign of an iron defiency. Most cravings however, are for strange combinations of food. We've all heard about the "pickles and ice cream" syndrome, and if you get hit at 2 am with such a craving, you probably aren't going to analyze the reason why. But do realize a craving is usually your body being off balance; your blood sugars may have dropped suddenly or your body fluids may not be in adequate balance. The goal is to not be overtaken by such demands but instead prevent them by attempting to meet your body's needs daily. But if it happens, try to make the best of your cravings. If you crave ice cream, try one of the lower fat sorbets or frozen yogurts with some fresh fruit on top.

If you crave cereal, make it a whole grain one topped with fresh fruit and skim milk. If you just have to have a cookie, make sure you have it with 8 ounces of skim milk.

Healthy Goal: Try to have small meals evenly throughout the day and always have your carbohydrate with your protein.

Cooperation is doing something with a smile that you have to do anyway.

What about constipation?

Constipation is very common in pregnancy, especially during the early weeks and again toward the end. The same hormones that cause your blood sugars to fluctuate also control the rate in which foods move through your digestive tract. This can result in major problems with constipation and gas formation unless you help your gastro-intestinal tract speed things up. Fiber and water act like a sponge in your digestive tract and help your food pass more easily.

Be sure to get plenty of whole grain carbohydrates, specifically unprocessed wheat bran, fresh fruits and leafy vegetables. Be sure to drink adequate water (8 oz. before and after every meal and snack) You might try filling a 2 quart container with water each morning and be sure it's gone by bedtime.

Also, exercise, especially walking, on a daily basis, will help keep the digestive tract moving. Just a 15 minute walk each day will do a world of good!

Healthy Goal: Laxatives aren't a healthy way to get rid of anything; fiber, water and exercise are.

What About Hemorrhoids?

Hemorrhoids are the result of the increased pressure on the veins of the rectal area (the equivalent of varicose veins in your legs).

For relief (1) Don't get constipated. Drink lots of water, increase your fiber and exercise. (2) A special help is to lie on your _left_ side for about 20 minutes every 4 to 6 hours. By doing this, you decrease pressure on the main vein draining the lower half of the body. (3) A dab of witch hazel works wonders. Take a cotton ball, soak it in cold witch hazel and apply it against your hemorrhoids until it's no longer cold, then repeat.

What about Heartburn?

The hormonal changes in pregnancy cause the emptying time of the stomach to slow and the sphincter between the esophagus and the stomach to stay more relaxed than normal, allowing a tendency for the acid in the stomach to be forced back into the esophagus. All of these changes may cause heartburn. It can be controlled by eating in an evenly distributed way through the day, helping to keep gastric acids neutralized. Do not resort to antacids! Remember to eat to _prevent_ heartburn, rather than trying to treat it once it's started.

There are some specific foods that aggravate heartburn by stimulating acid secretion: caffeine, pickled

92

foods, chili powder, pepper and peppermint candy. Orange juice and tomato sauces are major problems for many and are the first things to avoid if heartburn is chronic. Heartburn may also be caused by eating too fast. We aren't just a fast food generation, we're a fast eating one too. Heartburn can also be aggravated by excessive sugar or fat.

Healthy Goal: Prevent heartburn by avoiding certain specific foods that tend to cause it and eat slowly. At this time, be sure to drink lots of water but after meals, not on an empty stomach.

Friends are family you can choose for yourself.

The test of our love for God is the love we have for one another.

What About Exercise?

Keeping active while you are pregnant can be as beneficial to you psychologically as it is physically. Labor and delivery are stressful and require a lot from your body. It will be more comfortable for you if you have good muscle tone. Also, you will probably get back into shape faster and more easily if you've kept your body in good condition during your pregnancy.

Fitness should be a way of life for women of all ages but during pregnancy, special consideration is needed. You must remember that a pregnant woman is physically different.

The American College of Obstetricians and Gynecologists recommends walking, swimming, stationary cycling and modified forms of dancing and calisthenics as ideal forms of exercise for pregnant women as long as their pulse rate does not exceed 140 beats a minute and strenuous activity is not engaged in for more than 15 minutes. During normal pregnancy, maternal blood volume increases about 30% and heart rate and cardiac output are significantly elevated. The increased blood volume, coupled with the additional weight gain, cause a pregnant woman to reach her target rate with less vigorous activity than when not pregnant.

Excess heat should be avoided and and specifically avoid hot tubs, whirlpools, or steam rooms because they heat up the core temperature quickly.

Most doctors place restrictions on exercises with high risk of falling such as horseback riding, skiing, and skating. Sports involving balance may increase risk during pregnancy because of the altered center of gravity. Also avoid any work so strenuous that it competes with the baby for oxygen. Ask your doctor for the body building exercises specifically recommended during pregnancy for muscle strength and flexibility.

Walking can be your first step toward a lifetime of fitness. It's something we all know how to do, you can do anywhere and the only equipment you need is a comfortable pair of shoes. Many pregnant women have reported that their appetites decrease, they sleep better, and their general sense of well-being improves after making walking a part of their daily routine. Exercise and good nutrition are a dynamic duo for a healthy pregnancy.

You may experience small uterine contractions during or after aerobic exercise, but this is normal. You should stop exercising if it causes bleeding, painful cramping, nausea or shortness of breath. Discuss any problems with your doctor. If you are already involved in a fitness program, you should consult with your physican about any guidelines he would like for you to follow. Research shows there are many advantages to be gained from exercise.

What about swelling?

Swelling, or edema, is normal during pregnancy and is caused by the increased amount of fluid in your bloodstream. It's more noticable in the ankles and feet because the baby's weight puts pressure on the veins in your pelvis, slowing down the flow of blood from the legs to the heart. At times, however, the swelling may seem excessive, and may cause a sudden, unexplained jump in weight. In non-pregnant women, fluid retention is often caused by too high an intake of salt. In pregnancy, excessive swelling is more often caused by inadequate protein intake. Be sure you are eating 2 oz. of high quality, low fat protein every 2½ to 3 hours all through the day! Although salt used to be a

97

no-no for pregnant ladies, we now know that excess fluid retention is not usually caused by a <u>normal</u> salt (sodium chloride) intake, in fact, you require some sodium during pregnancy! <u>Don't restrict your fluid, don't take a diuretic (unless your doctor prescribes it), and don't cut out all sodium.</u> Do avoid processed foods that are high in salt (chips, dips, salted nuts, luncheon meats, convenience foods). They are low in nutrition and are triple threats: high in salt, fats and calories! Learn to <u>shake the salt habit</u> and to <u>drink water</u>, the most perfect diuretic. Flush those kidneys with cool, clear water, not a harsh diuretic that flushes nutrients out with it.

If you do start to swell, try rest, rest, rest! Laying on your side or sitting with your feet propped up also helps.

What about Toxemia?

Toxemia, or preeclampsia, is a condition found only in pregnancy that consists of swelling, elevated blood pressure and the loss of protein in the urine. The cause is not fully understood but it appears that women who enter a pregnancy obese or underweight and malnourished are more likely to develop the symptoms. It only occurs in 7% of first pregnancies and even less in later ones.

The symptoms usually appear about half way through the pregnancy and could be related to inadequate protein or vitamin B-6 intake. If you develop toxemia or extreme swelling, be sure and pay special attention to your protein intake. Good sources of protein are listed on page 22, and be sure you have it every

2½ hours with a whole grain carbohydrate all through the day and evening.

You should carefully avoid excessive salt intake. Bedrest is vitally important; resting 1 to 2 hours each day lying on your side will greatly help with the swelling and your whole feeling of well-being.

<u>Healthy Goal</u>: During this time of great nutritional needs, carefully follow the Ten Commandments of a Healthy Pregnancy meal plan.

Don't just live and let live but live and help live.

Religion may not keep you from sinning but it takes the joy out of it.

What about sleep?

The lowered metabolic rate of the first months of pregnancy may result in an increased need for sleep. You should attempt to get at least 8 hours of sleep a night, and don't feel guilty about taking a short nap during the day; this will not be easy to do once the baby arrives. You may find your sleep patterns changing in the final months, as many women seem to require less sleep. Listen to your body, and understand that adequate rest is a major part of wellness.

If you find yourself waking up during the night, and sleeping restlessly, be sure that you have a bedtime snack that will keep your blood sugar levels more even as you sleep. An ideal snack is a whole grain cereal with lowfat milk.

push *pull* *kick* *kick*

101

If you have difficulty going to sleep at night, be sure to get adequate exercise during the day; an evening walk followed by a warm shower does wonders! Also, be sure that you position yourself with lots of pillows for maximum comfort. Many women find that sleeping on their side with a pillow between their knees is a very comfortable position.

What about gas?

This is a natural by-product of a slower movement of food and waste through the system. If you are having a problem, try 1- Add small amounts of wheat bran to your cereal or other foods. Drink-<u>lots</u> of water to activate the fiber. (See Commandment 4 on page 28) 2. Certain foods are naturally gas forming: melons, cabbage, cauli-flower, broccoli, Brussels sprouts, iceberg lettuce, legumes. You don't have to avoid them but eat them at different times and in smaller portions. 3- Exercise helps to speed up the G.I tract motility and digestion. Walking can do wonders for you!

What about vegetarians and pregnancy?

The vegetarian diet can be a wonderfully nutritious and well balanced way of eating during pregnancy. It is especially easy for a "lacto-ovo" vegetarian (one who eats dairy foods and eggs) as the proteins in this diet are high quality substitutes for meat and fish.

The pregnant "vegan", (one who avoids <u>all</u> animal products) must take special care in planning her diet to get enough calories and to properly combine plant proteins to get all the essential amino acids (grains with legumes or seeds with legumes.) The vegan should also supplement with B-12 as it is not present in plant foods.

Getting proper amounts of high-iron foods should be a priority of both types of vegetarianism. A consult with a registered dietitian may be advised to aid in the careful planning of this special diet for a perfect pregnancy.

What about the teenage mom?

The pregnant teenager has an extra-special need for healthy food due to the extra high demands pregnancy places on her body.

The teenage years are a time to complete growth and development and to rebuild body stores of nutrients used during the changes of puberty. This rebuilding time will continue for 4 years after menstruation begins. Becoming pregnant during this time will put the body at high risk for health problems because the nutrient stores will not be replenished. There is a greater risk of delivering a premature, unhealthy or underweight baby as well as a greater tendency for the mom to develop toxemia and anemia. Read page 49 for the nutritional strategy to prevent anemia.

Eating the right thing at the right time can make the difference! It is a time to throw off the erratic dieting of teenage years and to focus on healthy eating. The pregnant teenager needs to eat for _her_ still growing body as well as the baby. She must be very careful to eat good whole grain carbohydrates balanced with 2 to 3 ounces of protein every 2½ to 3 hours through the day and evening. She will need 5 servings of high calcium foods each day and lots and lots of those darkly colored fruits and vegetables (6 servings a day) with 2 servings each day that are high in vitamin C.

Healthy goal: Teenage moms have a lot to gain from a good diet – and a lot to lose from a bad one! Realize how critical it is for you and that sweet baby you are nurturing for you to eat in a healthy way.

<u>What about Multiple Births</u>?

No one can begin to track the intense and wide gambit of emotions that are experienced with the news of a pregnancy. The news of "more than one" is just that much more powerful!

The physical needs of a multiple pregnancy are powerful as well. The requirement for vitamins and minerals increases, with a particularly high need for iron, calcium and folic acid. A supplement of these is usually given in addition to the prenatal vitamin and mineral. The mom expecting twins -or more- needs to learn all about preventing anemia (see page 49) and should increase her intake of high calcium foods to 6 servings each day. She should also eat lots and lots of dark green leafy veggies.

Energy demands are particularly high with multiple pregnancies, so the need to eat evenly and properly through the day and evening is very important! Rest is also vital and definite rest periods with mom lying on her side will be prescribed early in the pregnancy to avoid early labor. An extra serving of carbohydrates and 1 more ounce of protein should be added to each meal in the healthy meal plan (page 13) and 2 glasses of lowfat milk or its equivalent should be added as a snack. Eating every 2½ hours will also keep the appetite in better control.

When the patter of little feet becomes a stampede, how much weight should I gain?

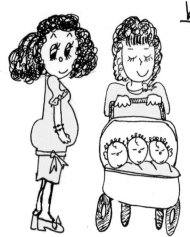

The total weight gain should be 35 to 37 pounds for twins; 38-40 pounds for triplets. Following the 10 Commandments of a Healthy Pregnancy will help you to keep a proper weight gain, stamina and energy.

Mothers are not for leaning on but to make leaning unnecessary.

Good health makes you feel now is the best time of year.

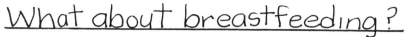

What about breastfeeding?

You may have noticed that your breasts are changing a great deal to prepare for feeding your baby after birth. Your breasts will enlarge and become fuller. Tenderness is normal. Veins become more noticeable under the skin and the nipple itself will darken and enlarge. You begin to produce a creamy-like fluid around the 4th month and may even notice some leakage. If so, just remove with warm water.

If you have chosen to breastfeed, begin now to prepare your nipples by exposing them to air and sunlight and by gently tugging and rolling nipples. You might try going braless around the house and gentle sunning braless through a window. Rubbing the nipples with a towel to toughen them is no longer advised as it removes the skin's natural protective qualities.

The decision to breast or bottlefeed your baby is not one that can be made under pressure. It is your decision. Read as much as you can about both so you can make the decision wisely. Your feelings will be sensed by your baby. This is your baby's most pleasurable time with you; make it enjoyable for both.

Breast milk is divinely created for your baby. It is perfectly sterile and digestable. It is convenient (no formula or bottles to prepare), it's perfect nutritionally and is always the right temperature. It provides substances that provide protection from infectious diseases and allergies.

Ninety nine percent of women who want to breast feed are physically able to do so. It does require time, patience and a good sense of humor. The greatest period of adjustment comes during the first 7 to 10 days.

Many people find a great deal of help and support from the La Leche League, an organization dedicated to assist the breast feeding mother. If you want to talk to someone when you're home, call your local chapter. They should be listed in your phone book.

The wonderful eating habits that allowed you to produce a healthy baby will allow you to produce healthy milk. Most important to your milk production and letdown reflex is your fluid intake. You will need 10 to 12 glasses of water each day. You may have to keep a chart; busy mothers forget fluids easily. Nothing will interfere with your milk production more. Another tip is to take a 16 oz. glass of water with you when you sit down to nurse and sip on it till it's gone. You will also need an extra serving of high-calcium food, 5 total each day. Start your morning feeding for the baby by drinking a glass of milk or fruit juice and cheese.

What do I take to the hospital?

You will want to have that suitcase all packed just waiting to go into labor. Many hospitals want you to bring the following items:

Two bras (nursing bras if you plan to breastfeed).

Robe and slippers

Nightgowns

Small amount of change for news papers, etc.

Personal items (toothpaste, tooth brush, cosmetics, hairbrush, deodorant, etc.)

Reading material

Watch or clock

Power Snacks, especially Trail Mix

Don't forget the baby's "going home" clothes

What about pre-pregnancy nutrition?

This is the day when many women are desperately trying to become pregnant. With the availability of modern tests and procedures, don't overlook the simple truth of preparing the body nutritionally. Eating well before pregnancy is much like building a home with a strong foundation, one that can strongly stand and house a very special guest.

If you are underweight, you should try to eat nutritiously to gain up to a healthy weight because women who weigh too little when they conceive are more likely to have smaller babies. Being underweight can also interfere with conception so ask your doctor for your ideal weight and for help in developing a nutritious mealplan.

113

If you are overweight, the time to lose the extra pounds is before pregnancy, not during. If you need to lose weight, it must be done in the most healthy way possible. Fad diets or starvation is no way to prepare your body for the big event, but good eating can cause you to lose weight as a side effect of proper nourishment.

Most women don't know that conception has taken place for 2 to 3 weeks. Those weeks are crucial, however, in the development of your baby. Now is the time to take a hard look at your intake of alcohol, caffeine and artificial sweeteners, drugs and smoking habits. Almost everything you swallow, inhale or inject can affect your baby. Make habit changes now before you conceive and your body is undergoing so many of its own physical changes.

<u>Healthy goal</u>: If you are trying to get pregnant now, treat your body as if you already are.

How does your baby grow?

The first moments: Conception usually occurs about 2 weeks after the beginning of the last menstrual cycle. After ovulation, the egg passes from an ovary into the Fallopian tube which is about 5 inches long. There is where the egg is joined by the sperm. It then travels to the uterus where it implants in the uterine wall, which usually takes 9 to 10 days. Your precious baby is beginning to grow rapidly, doubling in size every 24 hours.

Only 20 days after conception, the foundation for the child's brain, spinal cord and entire nervous system will have been established as well as rudiments of the eyes. The s-shaped, primitive heart is beginning to beat. Your baby to be is now 1/12 inch long and 1/6 inch wide.

Seventh week: The chest and abdomen are completely formed. The mouth opens; there are tiny shell-like external ears. All of the backbone is laid down and the spinal canal is closed over. Arms and legs are beginning to be visible. The baby is now ½ inch long and weighs 1/1000 of an ounce. What you eat is <u>so</u> important to your health and your baby's development!

<u>Eighth week:</u> The embryo is now a fetus to your doctor. It is "mama's precious" to you. Color begins to appear in the eyes, jaws are now formed and so are the teeth. Fingers and toes are present. The baby is about an inch long and weighs 1/30 ounce - less than an aspirin tablet.

<u>Twelfth week</u>: Your precious bundle of joy is now 3 inches long and weighs one whole ounce. Arms, legs, hands, feet, fingers and toes are fully formed. Nails appear. The brain, spinal cord and muscles connect and the baby can kick those tiny legs even though the movement can not be felt yet. That sweet thing can make a fist, open its mouth and squint those eyes.

116

Fourth month: Your precious baby you are nurturing is now 8 inches long and weighs 6 oz. The heartbeat is strong and audible with a stethoscope. At this time the baby may occupy the time by sucking its thumb. The skin is forming into several layers and is pink and wrinkled. The skeletal system is thickening and developing and some digestion even begins this month. The uterus is greatly enlarging.

Fifth month: The angel is 10 to 12 inches long and weighs 14 to 16 ounces. We finally got up to a pound. The baby is active now and you may begin to feel the movement, known as "quickening" at about 20 weeks. A covering like peach fuzz appears over the entire body and hair begins to grow. Internal organs are developing at an astonishing speed.

117

Sixth month:

Your angel now has finger and foot prints as the ridges on palms and soles of feet are fully formed. It has now grown to a length of 14 inches, weighs 2 pounds which means you will gain slightly more weight than previously. You will be able to feel definite little friendly kicks. The baby now makes you aware of its presence! A coating has formed called "vernix caseosa" to protect the skin from constant contact with the amniotic fluid. This vernix remains on the skin and serves as a lubricant during delivery as the baby passes through the birth canal. The eyes are open now and the baby can hear sounds.

Seventh month:

The weight of your child has doubled since last month. Skin is red and wrinkled but the fatty tissue begins to form underneath it and will fill it out to make it "soft as a baby's bottom."

118

The baby is gaining about ½ pound a week now and by the end of this month will weigh 2½ to 3½ pounds. and will be about 16 inches long. The organ that develops in these last months is the brain. Brain size increases tremendously and develops into a mature brain. Your nutrition during these last months greatly affects birth weight and brain size. If born now, the baby could probably survive with special neo-natal care as the organ systems are well developed. However, the next 2 months are periods of growth to ensure adequate size for a healthy full term delivery. It is also laying up stores of iron so be very careful that you avoid "empty calorie" foods.

Eight month: As more fat is deposited under the skin, the baby reaches about 5 pounds in weight and 18 inches in length. Lungs develop strength. Soon you will hear that wailing you've 119 been waiting for. The brain continues its rapid development, with the cells multiplying at a rapid rate. This continues to be a period of vital nutrient supply for the baby.

Ninth month: By delivery time your baby will weigh an average of 7 pounds and measure 20 to 21 inches long. Your baby's biggest weight gain will occur during this last month. It will store iron, fat soluble vitamins and minerals as reserves after birth, and also is building up immunities. That little darling is now ready and waiting to join its family.

Children have more need of models than critics.

A father is a man who expects his children to be as good as he meant to be.

Alive
And Well
In the
Fast Lane!

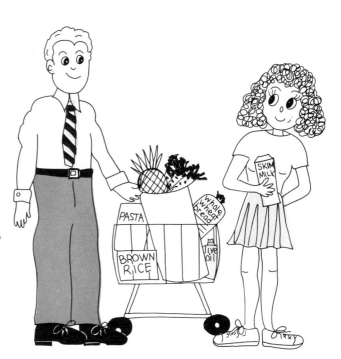

Your survival kit for staying Alive and Well in the Fast Food Lane!

SURVIVAL TIPS

You must be aware of the "hidden fats" in restaurant prepared foods and must never be timid about ordering foods in a "special style." You are paying (and paying well!) for the meal and service, and <u>deserve</u> to have foods prepared the way you desire. You also deserve to know the "content" of what you are going to eat! LEARN TO BE DISCRIMINATING, NOT INTIMIDATED!

1. Think BEFORE you order!

2. Order meats, fish or poultry broiled or grilled without butter, sauces <u>on the side</u>. Good choices: petite filet, marinated breast of chicken, broiled fish or seafood, and steamed shellfish.

3. Entrees that are poached in wine or lemon juice are acceptable as well as those simmered in tomato sauces.

4. When fresh vegetables are available, order them steamed without sauces or butter.

5. You may also have a slice of bread, a side order of pasta or a dinner roll as your complex carbohydrate.

122

6. A baked potato is the best choice for your carbohydrate, even a better choice than the rice pilaf that is usually sauteed in fat. (Ask for a substitution.) Ask for sour cream or butter <u>on the side.</u> A side dish of pasta with red sauce is a refreshing alternative to the potato; watch your portion.

7. Fresh fruit is a good substitution for your cooked vegetables (sometimes difficult to get in a restaurant). Fruit is many times served as an appetizer but they will serve it as dessert. (It is a much healthier choice than mousse!)

8. All salads must have dressing <u>on the side</u>! If you use dressing, lightly use 1 Tbsp. for taste with additional vinegar and lemon juice for moistness.

9. Remember to always have a carbohydrate and a protein source, never just a salad alone. You may order a chef's salad with extra turkey rather than ham, or a shrimp cocktail with your salad, just be sure to provide yourself with a protein. Many salad bars have a protein source in cottage cheese, grated cheese, or chopped eggs. Your carbohydrate may be a roll, crackers or baked potato.

10. Never eat all you can eat at all-you-can-eat brunches, restaurants, or covered dish dinners. Your overeating ("I want to get my money's worth") is not going to cheat the restaurant out of anything, but can cheat you out of many healthy years!

11. Menus are filled with clues about what their foods contain. AVOID THESE WORDS:

A LA MODE (with ice cream)
AU FROMAGE (with cheese)
AU GRATIN (in cheese sauce)
AU LAIT (with milk)
BASTED (with extra fat)
BISQUE (cream soup)
BUTTERED (with extra fat)
CASSEROLE (with extra fat)
CREAMED (with extra fat)
CRISPY (means fried)
ESCALLOPED (with cream sauce)
PAN-FRIED (fried with extra fat)
HASH (with extra fat)
HOLLANDAISE (with cream sauce)
SAUTEED (fried with extra fat)

If you see these words in the description of an appealing entree, be bold enough to ask for the entree prepared in a special way, i.e. if the description says "Buttered," ask for it without added butter; if the description says "Pan-Fried," ask for it grilled or poached instead.

12. Remember, it's your money, your health, and your waistline! Speak up. Don't be intimidated!

124

SOME SUGGESTIONS FOR DINING OUT HEALTHFULLY

MEXICAN — always order <u>ala carte</u> (refried beans are made with pure lard). Order a salad to be served immediately with dressing on the side. The salad will prevent "eat because they're there" munching on the chips. And beware of the Margaritas—they are loaded with both salt and sugar, to say nothing of the alcohol!

Ideas: Black Bean Soup, Chili, or Gazpacho, Chicken Burrito,
Tostada, or Enchilada, Soft Chicken Tacos,
Chicken Fajitas (without added fat)

ORIENTAL — order dishes that have been <u>lightly</u> stir fried (not deep fried like egg rolls) without heavy gravies or sweet and sour sauces. Eat <u>1/2 portion</u> served with <u>steamed</u> rice; do not use fried. Many restaurants will prepare food without MSG if you ask, and be careful to watch the soy sauce you add. Both are loaded with sodium! All items can be acceptable for the bold sodium watcher who asks for neither soy sauce nor MSG!

Ideas: Bamboo-steamed vegetables with chicken, seafood or fish
Moo Goo Gai Pan, Shrimp or Tofu with vegetables (with no MSG and little oil)
Wonton, hot and sour or miso soup, Udon with meat and vegetables

ITALIAN - portion size control is important here; the typical plate full of spaghetti is 5 times too much!! You will do much better with a side dish or appetizer portion. Always order salad with dressing on the side, and never hesitate to ask for a red sauce rather than a butter or white sauce.

Ideas:
*Lasagna (have approximately a 3" x 5" piece)
Canneloni
*Grilled chicken with pasta side dish or bread
*Fresh fish with pasta side dish or bread
*Clams Linquine with Red Sauce (careful with amounts of pasta eaten!)
*Minestrone Soup and Salad, dressing on side; ala carte mozzarella cheese or meatballs for protein.
*Side dish of spaghetti with 2 ala carte meatballs
*Grilled Shrimp on Fettucine with Red Sauce

*Lower sodium choice - have with slice of bread rather than pasta with red sauce.

STEAK HOUSES - Portion control is also crucial here. A 16 oz. steak or prime rib will give you 5 times more than needed. Order the smallest cut available and don't be fearful of taking some home! Lowest sodium choice is filet or london broil without salt.

Ideas:
Petite Cut Filet, Shish-Ka-Bob or Brochette
Slices of London Broil (no sauces, please!)
Hawaiian Chicken, Charbroiled Shrimp

126

SEAFOOD - order fish/seafood when possible, steamed, boiled, grilled or broiled <u>without butter</u>. A small amount of cocktail sauce is a better choice for dipping than butter (2 dips in butter = 50 calories). Remember small seafood items such as shrimp, oysters etc. are "deadly" in terms of fat and calories when fried; the surface area is so high, more breading adheres and absorbs more fat. All can be low sodium choices when grilled and if sauces are avoided.

Ideas: Fresh Fish of the Day - Grilled when possible, without butter and sauce to the side
Steamed oysters, shrimp, or clams (5 = 1 oz. protein)
Lobster/Crabmeat/Crab Claws (1/4 cup = 1 oz. protein)
Seafood Kabobs, Mesquite grilled shrimp
Blackened Fish prepared without butter (high sodium)

APPETIZER HEAVENS - Many restaurants specialize in appetizers: Fried Cheese, Nachos, Fried Potato Skins "loaded" with bacon, sour cream and cheese, fried zucchini and mushrooms. These are cardiovascular nightmares when you consider 2 potato skins OR 2 pieces of fried cheese are basically the fat calories of a whole meal (and should be used as such!). Many restaurants are offering raw vegetable platters; vegetables are safe but not the dip, so very, very carefully indulge!

Good choices: Chicken burritos or fajitas, Grilled Seafood
Marinated chicken breast, Non-creamed Soup

HEALTH/NATURAL FOOD RESTAURANTS - do not feel "safe" here <u>by any means!</u> Although you will have an opportunity to get whole grains and nicer fresh vegetable salads, the fats and sodium come in even more deceptively! Beware of sauces and high fat cheeses smothering the foods, and high fat dressings on salads and sandwiches. Many foods are prepared in the same way as at the Fast Food Restaurant, they just have healthier sounding names. You can do well here, however, with judicious choices. Again, the salads and salad bars are lovely, just follow the same guideline of dressing to the side and its minimal use. If you have a cheese dish, be sure to use no other added fats in the meal; the cheese will contain enough for the day!

Good choices: Vegetable Soup and 1/2 sandwich (avoid tuna/chicken salad due to mayo)
"Chef" type salad and whole grain roll (no ham)
Stir fry dishes asking for "light" on oil
Marinated breast of chicken
Fresh fish of the day - grilled when possible
Vegetable Omelet with whole grain roll
Pitas stuffed with vegetables and cheese
Fruit plate with plain yogurt/cottage cheese and whole grain roll

128

BREAKFAST OUT — Breakfast can be a special meal out due to such safe and easy choices. If breakfast is later than normal, have a snack when first arising, then the later meal. You also may choose to have your larger lunch portions for breakfast, and a smaller lunch 3 to 4 hours later. Follow these guidelines in ordering:

1. Be sure to always order whole wheat toast or grits unbuttered; you may add one teaspoon of butter, if desired.

2. You are usually safer to order a la carte so that you are not paying for, or tempted by, the abundance of food in the "breakfast specials" or buffets.

3. Be bold and creative in ordering! Rather than accepting French toast with syrup and bacon; ask for it made with whole wheat bread, no syrup and a side dish of fresh berries or fruit instead. Many restaurants will substitute cottage cheese or 1 egg for the meat. Many restaurants also serve oatmeal and cereal even though it's not always on the menu. It's a nice carbohydrate with milk and fresh fruit, especially strawberries or blueberries.

4. Always look for a protein and a carbohydrate source. A Danish doesn't do it!

> **Good choices:** Eggs and whole wheat toast or English muffin
> French Toast with berries
> Fresh vegetable omelet and toast
> Cereal with skim milk and fruit
> Fresh fruit bowl with cottage cheese and
> whole wheat toast

HEALTHIER "FAST FOOD"

As in any experience with dining out, the healthy "fast food gourmet" must be aware of the hidden fats in foods ordered.

* SPECIAL SAUCES: "NOT-SO-SPECIAL" FAT AND SODIUM! It's the mayonnaise, special sauces, sour cream, etc. that triples the fat, sodium and calories in fast foods; always order your food without them!

* Stuffed potatoes may seem a healthy addition to the fast food menu but not with the cheese sauces they are smothered in — equivalent to 9 PATS OF BUTTER PER POTATO! Ask for grated cheese with no butter, instead.

* Chicken is truly a lowfat alternative over beef, but not when it's batter fried! One serving of chicken nuggets has the equivalent of five pats of butter, over twice of what you would get in a regular hamburger. And the fat it's soaked in is purely saturated, largely melted beef fat. A chicken sandwich is no health package either. This greasy sandwich has enough fat to equal 11 pats of butter, unless the chicken is grilled.

* Croissant Sandwiches aren't a whole lot more than "breakfast on a grease bun"! Most of the croissants have the equivalant of more than 4.5 pats of butter and the toppings add insult to injury!

* Salad bars can be a good way to add fiber and nutrients to a meal, but it's only the salad vegetables that do so. The mayonnaise based salads, the croutons, and the bacon bits should be left on the bar, and dressing used sparingly. Use less dressing with extra lemon juice or vinegar for moistness.

* Frozen yogurt, although lower in fat and cholesterol, contains more sugar than ice cream - so it is <u>not</u> a perfectly healthy substitute. This also applies to the frozen Tofu desserts. Look for some of the new sorbet-like frozen desserts that are primarily fruit. They will contain some sugar, but usually not in such high amounts.

Stop! Don't get discouraged and think you can't ever eat fast foods and still be healthy! You can have a healthy fast food meal, but you must learn to make good choices. The trick is to learn what you CAN eat and then think positively. Rather than feeling dismayed about everything you can't order, use your creativity and knowledge to find things you can.

The man who believes he can do something is probably right, and so is the man who believes he can't.

BURGER KING
Hamburger Deluxe (no mayo!) - for women
Whopper (no mayo!) - for men
(A chicken sandwich has enough fat to equal 11 pats of butter!)
B.K. Broiler Chicken Sandwich (without dressing or mayo!)
Chunky Chicken Salad

MCDONALDS
Quarter pounder
Oriental Chicken Salad; crackers for complex carbohydrate

Chunky Chicken Salad (with your own whole grain, low salt crackers
for carbohydrate) and Lite Vinaigrette Dressing

Hamburger (small)
McLean Deluxe Sandwich (no mayo)
Chicken Fajitas

WENDY'S
Stuffed Potatoes - (plain without cheese sauce; get with chili instead)
Salad Bar - use raw vegetables as desired (avoid potato salad,
macaroni salad, and so forth; use garbanzo beans or chili for protein)
Single Hamburger on bun, without mayo
Caesar Side Salad (without dressing)
Grilled Chicken Sandwich

132

WENDY'S (continued)
Baked Potato (plain, without cheese sauce; get with chili instead)
Jr. Hamburger (without mayo)

HARDEE'S
Chicken 'n' Pasta Salad
Grilled Chicken Sandwich (no mayo!)
Hamburger (no mayo)

STEAK 'N SHAKE
Steakburger (no mayo!)
3-Way Chili

CHICK-FIL-A
Grilled Chicken Salad (no-oil salad dressing)
Grilled Chicken Sandwich (no mayo!)

TACO BELL
Soft Taco (chicken)
Taco, hardshell (chicken)
Fiesta Tostada

DAIRY QUEEN
BBQ Beef Sandwich
Grilled Chicken Fillet Sandwich (no sauce!)

ARBY'S OR RAX
Arby's Roast Beef or Chicken Sandwich (no mayo!)
Rax Turkey (no mayo!)
Roast Beef Sandwich (no sauce)
Arby's Fajita Pita

PIZZA PLACES
Personal-size cheese pizza, with vegetables if desired (eat three quarters and save the remaining quarter for a snack)
Thin crust 13" (medium) cheese pizza with vegetables if desired (no sausage or pepperoni) 2 slices for women; 3 slices for men

SUB SHOPS OR DELI
Mini-sub (turkey, roast beef no oil or mayo)
Snack sub - 6 inches (turkey, roast beef cheese no oil or mayo)
Avoid Tuna subs - loaded with fat!
Deli and grocery stores will usually make you turkey, roast beef or Jarlsberg Lite sandwiches (ask for 3 ounces of meat on sandwich).

Menus
and
Recipes

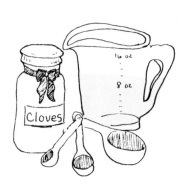

PERFECT BREAKFASTS
THAT ARE QUICK, EASY AND DELICIOUS!

Remember — breakfast is the "stick" that stokes your metabolic fire. You need more than just a piece of toast and coffee to give your baby a "Sunny Beginning." Try the following breakfast ideas, a different one every day, for a wonderful variety of ways to start your day just right!

1) **CHEESE DANISH**

1 whole wheat English muffin
2 oz. light or no fat cream cheese
2 Tbsp. raisins OR all fruit preserves

Spread muffin with light or no fat cream cheese; if possible, warm in toaster oven. Top with raisins or preserves. (Another marvelous choice:
mash 1/4 cup fresh berries and put on top of cheese and muffin.)
Makes 1 serving.

2 Complex CHO: Muffin / 2 oz. Protein: Cheese
1 Simple CHO: Raisins

2) OATMEAL WITH A DIFFERENCE

2/3 cup of old fashioned Oats
1 cup skim milk
1/2 cup unsweetened apple juice

1 Tbsp. raisins
cinnamon
1/2 tsp. vanilla

Bring milk, apple juice and oatmeal to a boil. Gently cook for 5 minutes, stirring occasionally. Add raisins, vanilla and cinnamon; let sit covered for 2-3 minutes to thicken.

Makes 1 serving.

2 Complex CHO: Oats / 2 oz. Protein: Milk
1 Simple CHO: Juice and Raisins

3) PEANUT BUTTER DANISH

1 slice 100% whole grain bread
1 Tbsp. natural peanut butter

1/2 banana
8 oz. skim milk

Slice banana lengthwise and place with inside facing down on the slice of bread. Top with peanut butter. Broil until peanut butter is slightly brown and bubbly. Surprise! Have with an 8 oz. glass of skim milk. Makes 1 serving.

2 Complex CHO: Bread / Protein: Peanut Butter and milk
1 Simple CHO: Banana

4) **SUNDAY FRENCH TOAST** *You can freeze the extras and pop them in the toaster on a busy morning.*

6 egg whites, lightly beaten
1 tsp. vanilla
1-1/2 cups skim milk
1/2 tsp. cinnamon
6 slices whole wheat bread
Fruit Preserves (no sugar) or mashed fresh fruit

Beat together egg whites, milk, vanilla and cinnamon. Add bread slices one at a time, letting the bread absorb liquid in the process. May let sit for a few minutes. Spray non-stick skillet with cooking spray and heat. Gently lift the bread with spatula into skillet and cook until golden brown on each side. Serve topped with 1/2 cup fresh fruit or 1 Tbsp. (no sugar) preserves.
Makes 2 servings.

2 Complex CHO: Bread / 2 oz. Protein: Eggs, Milk
1 Simple CHO: Fruit

Add the juice of half an orange and it's even better!

137

5) **PERFECT BOWL OF CEREAL**

1-1/2 cups approved cereal
1-1/2 cups skim milk
1 Tbsp. unprocessed wheat bran AND 1 Tbsp. oat bran
1/2 cup fruit OR 1 small banana OR 2 Tbsp. raisins (1 tiny box)

APPROVED CEREALS: Kellogg's Nutrigrain (all types), Grapenuts (only use 1/4 cup, however), Shredded Wheat, Shredded Wheat-N-Bran, Puffed Wheat, Puffed Rice, oatmeal, Wheatena, Raisin Squares, Oat Bran, Muesli.

2 Complex CHO: Cereal / 2 oz. Protein: Milk
1 Simple CHO: Fruit

6) **BREAKFAST SHAKE**

1/2 cup frozen fruit*   **2 Tbsp. nonfat dry milk**
1 cup skim milk   **2 Tbsp. wheat germ**
1 tsp. vanilla   **2 tsp. oat bran**

Blend frozen fruit in blender. Add remaining ingredients and continue blending till smooth.

1 Complex CHO: Wheat Germ and Bran / 2 oz. Protein: Milk
1 Simple CHO: Fruit

*Don't throw away your very ripe bananas. Peel and freeze in freezer bags and use for your shakes.

138

7) **BREAKFAST PARFAIT**

1 cup plain, nonfat yogurt
1/2 cup blueberries OR 1 small mashed banana OR 1/2 cup unsweetened crushed pineapple
    (strawberries are too tart)
1 Tbsp. all fruit preserves
1/2 cup Grapenuts
cinnamon

Layer parfait style into tall parfait glass yogurt, fruit and cereal. Sprinkle with cinnamon and ENJOY!

2 Complex CHO: Cereal / 2 oz. Protein: Yogurt
1 Simple CHO: Fruit

8) **CHEESE APPLE SURPRISE**

2 slices whole wheat bread   **1/2 apple, thinly sliced**
1 Tbsp. raisins   **2 oz. mozzarella cheese**

Top bread with apple and raisins. Place cheese on apple-raisin layer. Broil until cheese is bubbly.
Makes 1 serving.

2 Complex CHO: Bread / 2 oz. Protein: Cheese
1 Simple CHO: Apple and Raisins

9) **MUFFIN MAGIC**

Apple Date Muffins (your complex carbohydrate) - page 172
1-1/2 cups Skim Milk or Plain, Nonfat Yogurt (your protein)
Fresh Fruit (your simple carbohydrate)

WONDERFUL LUNCHES

Don't skip lunch, and don't get into a rut either! For a lunch that will refresh you and keep your energy high, try one of these delicious and fast complete meals.

1) <u>SEAFOOD SALAD</u>

3/4 cup waterpacked tuna or salmon
1 tsp. Dijon mustard
1 Tbsp. reduced calorie mayonnaise
8 seasoned Ry-Krisp

1 stalk chopped celery
1/4 tsp. beau monde (optional)
1/4 tsp. dill
pepper to taste

Mix together ingredients. Serve on bed of torn romaine lettuce with 10 whole grain crackers and fresh fruit.

Complex CHO: Crackers / Protein: Fish
Simple CHO: Fruit / Added Fat: Mayonnaise

2) <u>PEANUT BUTTER AND BANANA SANDWICH</u>

1 Tbsp. natural peanut butter (never, never commercial)
2 slices of whole wheat bread
1 small sliced banana
8 oz. skim milk

Make sandwich with bread, peanut butter and sliced banana.
Have with 8 oz. skim milk.

Complex CHO: Bread / Protein: Peanut Butter and Milk
Simple CHO: Banana

140

3) CHEF'S SALAD

As many sliced veggies as possible (try to have at least 5)
romaine lettuce
3 oz. chicken, turkey or Alpine Lace "Lean and Free"

Toss vegetables with lettuce; top with meat or cheese. You may use croutons made by toasting 2 pieces whole wheat that have been sprinkled with garlic powder (not salt!). Cut these into cubes and store in jar or tin to have on hand. Serve with whole grain crackers and fresh fruit.

Complex CHO: Crackers/Croutons / Protein: Meat or Cheese
Simple CHO: Fruit / Added Fat: 1 Tbsp. Dressing

4) CHICKEN, TURKEY OR ROAST BEEF SANDWICH

3 oz. meat (trimmed of all fat)
2 slices whole wheat bread
1 tsp. mayonnaise and/or mustard
lettuce and sliced tomato

Spread bread with mayo and/or mustard. Layer with meat of choice; top with lettuce and tomato. Serve with a delicious piece of fruit.

Complex CHO: Bread / Protein: Turkey
Simple CHO: Fruit / Added Fat: Mayonnaise

141

5) CHICKEN OF THE LAND OR SEA APPLE SANDWICH

3/4 cup waterpacked tuna or chicken
1 small stalk of chopped celery
1 Tbsp. reduced calorie mayonnaise

1 small chopped apple
1 whole wheat pita
romaine lettuce leaves

Mix together first 4 ingredients. Stuff into 2 halved pita lined
with lettuce.

Complex CHO: Pita / Protein: Chicken
Simple CHO: Fruit / Added Fat: Mayonnaise

6) VEGGIE SANDWICH

1 whole wheat pita
3 oz. cheese (mozzarella, skimmed cheddar, or Alpine Lace "Lean and Free)
a few mushrooms and green pepper rings
sliced tomato

Stuff halved pita with 1 oz. cheese each and vegetables.
Microwave on high for 2 to 3 minutes. Add a couple of tomato
slices and be ready for a treat. Serve with a fruit juice spritzer
(1/2 cup juice mixed with club soda or seltzer) over ice.

Complex CHO: Pita / Protein: Cheese
Simple CHO: Juice

7) **HEALTHY HAMBURGER**

1 whole wheat hamburger bun
3 oz. uncooked ground round or ground turkey patty
lettuce and tomato slices

Grill or broil hamburger patty (the fat will drain through rack and will cook meat down to 3 oz.). Place on whole wheat bun with lettuce, tomato slices, mustard and a small amount of ketchup (if desired). 1 pound of ground round = 4 3 oz. patties after cooking. Serve with Melon Slices.

Complex CHO: Bun / Protein: Burger
Simple CHO: Melon

8) **CARROT-CHEESE MELT**

1 1/2 oz. grated carrots (about 1/2 cup)   **2 slices whole wheat bread**
1-1/2 oz. grated mozzarella cheese   **8 oz. skim milk**

Mix together carrots and cheese. Spread bread with carrot-cheese mix. Grill in teflon skillet till cheese melts. Add tomato slices, lettuce (and even alfalfa sprouts!).

Complex CHO: Bread / Protein: Cheese and Milk
Simple CHO: Carrots

143

EASY, DELICIOUS AND HEALTHY DINNERS

There are times that having a basic format to work from can be invaluable! These are eight meals that you can use as a beginning place: they are perfectly balanced, everyone will like them, and they are easy! Freeze properly portioned leftovers in freezer Zip Lock® bags for quick meals when you need them most!

1) **OVEN BAKED CHICKEN** — (your protein)
    PEAS ROSEMARY — (your complex carbohydrate)
    STEAMED CABBAGE — (your simple carbohydrate)
    CARROT-RAISIN SALAD — (the rest of your simple carbohydrate)

OVEN BAKED CHICKEN *It tastes like fried chicken!*

2 egg whites, lightly beaten
2 cups Nutrigrain Wheat cereal, crushed
1/4 tsp. pepper
6 chicken half-breasts, deboned and skinned

1 Tbsp. water
1/4 tsp. garlic powder
1/4 tsp. seasoned salt (optional)

Mix together egg and water in shallow dish; set aside. Combine crushed cereal and spices. Dip chicken in egg mixture, then dredge in cereal mixture, coating well. Arrange in baking pan coated with cooking spray. Bake, uncovered, at 350 degrees for 45 minutes, or until tender. Yields 6 servings, each giving you your protein and part of your complex carbohydrate.

PEAS ROSEMARY

1 pkg. frozen peas, cooked and drained
2 tsp. olive oil
2 cloves minced garlic
1/4 cup chopped onion
1/4 tsp. pepper
1 tsp. rosemary
1/4 tsp. salt (optional)

Saute garlic and onion in oil till tender. Add rosemary, salt and pepper and continue to saute one more minute. Toss with peas. Makes 4 servings; one serving would be your complex carbohydrate.

CARROT SALAD A LA DIFFERENCE

1 lb. coarsely grated carrots
2 medium apples, grated
1 cup firm plain nonfat yogurt
1/2 cup crushed unsweetened pineapple
1/2 cup raisins

Combine all ingredients and chill. Makes 12 servings; 1 cup serving counts as part of your simple carbohydrate.

2) **MARVELOUS MEATLOAF** — (your protein and part of your complex carbohydrates)
   CORN ON COB — (your complex carbohydrate)
   COLORFUL GREEN BEANS — (your simple carbohydrate)
   ROMAINE SALAD — (your healthy munchie)

MARVELOUS MEATLOAF

2 lbs. ground round or ground turkey
2 cups old fashioned oats
3/4 cup minced onion
1/4 green pepper, minced
2 eggs, slightly beaten

1/2 tsp. each salt and pepper
1 Tbsp. worcestershire sauce
1 tsp. dry mustard
1/4 cup skim milk
3/4 cup tomato sauce

In large bowl, mix together all ingredients except for 1/2 cup of the tomato sauce. Shape meat into 2 loaves and place in loaf pans sprayed with cooking spray. Spread the additional 1/2 cup tomato sauce on top. Bake in 400 degree oven for 40 minutes. A 3 oz. serving counts as your protein.

COLORFUL GREEN BEANS

1 lb. green beans
1/2 cup chopped onion
1/2 tsp. salt (optional)
2 medium tomatoes, peeled and cut into 8 wedges

1 tsp. olive oil
1/2 cup chopped celery
1/4 tsp. pepper

Remove strings from beans; wash and cut diagonally into 2" pieces. Heat oil in skillet, add onion and celery to skillet and saute until tender; add beans, salt and pepper. Cover and simmer 10 minutes, stirring occasionally. Add tomato; cover and cook an additional 5 minutes. Makes 4 servings; each serving counts as your simple carbohydrate.

3) **HAWAIIAN CHICKEN** — (your protein)
   WILD RICE PILAF — (your complex carbohydrate)
   GREEN BEANS AND MUSHROOMS — (your simple carbohydrate)
   SLICED TOMATOES — (your healthy munchie)

HAWAIIAN CHICKEN

1/3 cup unsweetened pineapple juice   **2 cloves garlic**
1/3 cup low sodium soy sauce   **1 Tbsp. parsley**
1/3 cup sherry or alcohol-free Chardonnay **ground pepper to taste**
4 skinned chicken breasts

Mix all but chicken. Marinate chicken breasts (skinned, deboned and split lengthwise) for 3-4 hours or overnight. (The marinade adds no significant calories.) Grill. Makes 4 servings; one serving would be your protein.

WILD RICE PILAF

1 tsp. olive oil
1 medium onion, chopped
1 clove minced garlic
1 stalk celery, chopped
2-1/3 cups chicken broth

1/4 cup wild rice
3/4 cup brown rice
1/4 tsp. salt (optional)
1 Tbsp. parsley

Saute vegetables in medium saucepan with 1 tsp. olive oil. Add broth and optional salt; bring to boil and add rices. Boil for one minute - reduce heat and simmer for 45 minutes until the liquid is absorbed. Garnish with parsley. Makes 6 half-cup servings; 1 cup would be your complex carbohydrate.

GREEN BEANS WITH MUSHROOMS

1 tsp. olive oil
1 clove minced garlic
1/2 lb. washed mushrooms
1/2 tsp. rosemary
1/2 tsp. basil

1 Tbsp. parsley
1/2 tsp. salt (optional)
1/4 tsp. pepper
1 lb. steamed green beans

Saute olive oil, garlic and mushrooms in non-stick pan for 3–4 minutes. Add spices and simmer covered for 1 more minute. Toss well with beans. Makes 4 servings; each counts as your simple carbohydrate.

4) **SALMON OF THE DAY** — (this is your protein)
   BAKED SWEET POTATO — (this is your complex carbohydrate)
   STEAMED BROCCOLI — (this is your simple carbohydrate)
   WALDORF SALAD — (this is your simple carbohydrate)

BAKED SALMON IN A POUCH

1/4 cup cider vinegar
1/2 tsp. Dijon mustard
1/2 tsp. dillweed
1/4 tsp. minced garlic

4 salmon steaks, 1" thick (approx. 1 lb.)
1 sliced green pepper
1 thinly sliced tomato
1 minced scallion

Combine vinegar, mustard, dill and garlic in glass baking dish. Add salmon and marinate for 10 minutes. Turn salmon over and marinate 10 minutes more. Cut 4 8" x 8" sheets of aluminum foil. For each serving, place a salmon steak in the center of foil. Distribute peppers, tomatoes and scallions on top. Drizzle with marinade. Fold and pinch foil to seal fish inside. Bake at 375 degrees for 15 to 20 minutes. Remove from foil and serve immediately. Makes 4 servings; each gives you protein.

Love is like the 5 loaves and 2 fishes. It doesn't start to multiply until you give it away.

POACHED SALMON

1-1/2 cups Chablis or other white wine
1 lemon, sliced
1 tsp. dried dillweed
1/4 tsp. pepper
4 salmon steaks, 1" thick (approx. 1 lb.)

1/2 cup water
1 onion, sliced
4 sprigs parsley
extra sliced lemon

Combine all ingredients except fish and additional lemon slices in a large skillet. Bring to a boil; cover, reduce heat, and simmer 5 minutes. Add salmon steaks or fillets; cover and simmer 8 minutes or until fish flakes easily. Remove from skillet; garnish with lemon slices. Makes 4 servings; each gives you protein.

GRILLED SALMON

1/2 tsp. allspice
1 tsp. cardamon (optional)
2 cloves garlic, minced

1/3 cup lime juice
1-1/3 lbs. salmon steaks, about 1" thick
additional lime slices

Combine spices with garlic and lime juice. Arrange salmon in a single layer in shallow dish; cover with marinade. Let stand for 15 minutes, then turn over and let stand for 15 minutes more. Grill salmon for 5 minutes per side or until it flakes easily. Makes 4 servings; 1 serving counts as protein.

SALMON LOAF

1 medium onion, chopped
3/4 cup old fashioned oats (uncooked)
1/2 cup unprocessed bran
15-1/2 oz. can salmon, drained
1 cup buttermilk
1/4 tsp. garlic powder

2 eggs, lightly beaten
1 Tbsp. parsley
1/2 tsp. dill
1/2 tsp. salt, if desired
1/4 tsp. pepper
lemon and parsley to garnish

Mix together all ingredients. Pack into an 8-1/2 x 4-1/2 inch bread pan sprayed with non-stick spray. Bake at 350 degrees for 40 minutes, until firm. Garnish with lemon wedges and parsley. Makes 6 servings; each serving counts as your protein and part of your complex carbohydrate.

WALDORF IN DISGUISE

2 large apples, in chunks
1/2 cup unsweetened pineapple chunks
1/2 stalk chopped celery
1/2 cup sliced carrot
2 Tbsp. chopped walnuts

1 sliced green pepper
1 small orange, sectioned
1/4 cup raisins
1-1/4 cups Orange Yogurt
     dressing

Combine apples, pineapple, celery, carrots, green pepper, orange and raisins. Add dressing, mixing well. Chill. Sprinkle with chopped nuts before serving. Makes 6 half-cup servings, each giving 2 servings of simple carbohydrates.

Dressing:

3/4 cup plain low-fat yogurt
juice from 1/2 lemon

1/2 cup orange juice
dash salt and cinnamon

*Mix a lot of dressing at one time and keep in refrigerator for a wonderful fruit topping

5) **CHILI CON CARNE** — (this is your protein, complex and simple carbohydrate)
   ROMAINE SALAD — (this is your healthy munchie)
   SLICED MELON — (this is more simple carbohydrate)

CHILI CON CARNE*

1 lb. ground round or ground turkey
2 tsp. olive oil
1 tsp. basil
2-3 tsp. chili powder
1 tsp. salt (optional)
1/8 tsp. pepper
1 medium can red kidney beans, drained and rinsed

28 oz. can undrained tomatoes
15-1/2 oz. can tomato sauce
1 cup chopped onion
2 cloves crushed garlic
1 cup chopped celery
3 cups green peppers, chopped

Place ground meat in hard plastic colander; place colander in glass bowl in microwave. Microwave on high for 3 minutes; break up. Continue cooking another 3 minutes, or until brown; stir again. In a 3-4 qt. sauce pan, heat oil and add 3/4 cup of the onions, the garlic, the celery, and 1 cup of the green peppers. Saute 5-8 minutes over moderate heat, stirring occasionally, until

152

tender. Add tomatoes, breaking them up as you stir them in. Stir in the browned meat, tomato sauce, chili powder, basil, salt and pepper. Cover and simmer 1 hour over low heat. Uncover and simmer 40-60 minutes longer, stirring occasionally to develop flavor. Stir in the beans and cook 5 minutes longer. Garnish with remaining onions and green peppers to make it pretty. 2 cups = 1 serving.

*May make this vegetarian by adding another can of kidney beans and serving over rice or pasta.

6) **CHICKEN OF THE DAY** — (your protein and your complex CHO)
   STEAMED ASPARAGUS — (counts as part of your simple CHO)
   SPINACH AND APPLE SALAD — (counts as health munchie and the meal's addedfat)

BASQUE CHICKEN

1 lg. green pepper, in strips	**1/2 tsp. salt (optional)**
2 med. onions, sliced and in rings	**1/4 tsp. black pepper**
1/4 lb. thinly sliced mushrooms	**1/4 tsp. cayenne**
2 cloves minced garlic	**1-1/2 cups tomato puree**
8 red potatoes, thinly sliced	**1/4 cup dry white wine**
2 tsp. cornstarch	**1 Tbsp. water**

2 chicken breasts, skinned, deboned and split lengthwise

Place vegetables in roasting pan. Place chicken pieces over vegetables; sprinkle with spices. Mix tomato puree and wine; pour into roasting pan. Bake at 375 degrees for 1 hour uncovered or until tender and browned. Pour cooking liquid with vegetables into skillet. Mix cornstarch and water; stir into skillet. Heat to boiling; cook, stirring constantly until thickened and clear. Pour sauce and vegetables over chicken and serve. This makes 4 servings; 1 piece of chicken counts as your protein, two potatoes count as your complex carbohydrate, and 1 cup sauce counts as your simple carbohydrate.

STIR FRY CHICKEN WITH SNOW PEAS

2 cloves garlic, minced
2 Tbsp. low sodium soy sauce
1 Tbsp. sherry
2 Tbsp. cornstarch
2 split chicken breasts, cut into 1 inch cubes

20 snow pea pods, sliced
1/2 cup water chestnut, drained
1/2 cup chicken stock
2 tsp. peanut or canola oil

Mix together garlic, soy sauce, sherry, and cornstarch; marinate chicken pieces in mixture for 15 minutes. Spray wok with non-stick cooking spray, then heat with 2 tsp. peanut oil. Add chicken; stir fry for 30 seconds. Add chicken broth; stir fry until thickened. Serve immediately. Wonderful over brown rice. Makes 2 servings; each gives 2-3 oz. protein, 1 simple carbohydrate and 1 added fat. The brown rice would be your complex carbohydrate.

Doing nothing is tiresome - you can't stop and rest.

SPINACH AND APPLE SALAD

1 Tbsp. canola oil
1-1/2 tsp. basil
1 tsp. onion powder
1/2 tsp. salt (optional)
1/8 tsp. pepper

3/4 cup apple juice
2 Tbsp. cider vinegar
4 cups spinach, torn in pieces
2 cups thinly sliced apple
1/2 cup orange segments

Prepare dressing: In small bowl, combine oil, basil, onion powder, salt and pepper; set aside 10 minutes for flavors to blend. Stir in apple juice and vinegar. In large bowl, combine spinach, apple and oranges. Toss with 1/2 cup dressing; serve immediately. Refrigerate remaining dressing for other salads or marinade. Makes 6 healthy munchie servings and 1 added fat/svg.

7) **ITALIAN SWISS STEAK** — (your protein)
   WHOLE WHEAT NOODLES — (your complex carbohydrate)
   STEAMED YELLOW SQUASH — (part of your simple carbohydrate)
   ROMAINE LETTUCE SALAD — (your healthy munchie)

ITALIAN SWISS STEAK

1 lb. lean round steak*, trimmed of fat
1/2 cup water
1 medium onion, thinly sliced
1 green pepper, thinly sliced
2 small tomatoes, cut in wedges
1/4 lb. mushrooms

1/2 tsp. basil
1/2 tsp. oregano
1 Tbsp. parsley
1/2 tsp. garlic powder
1/4 tsp. each salt and pepper

Brown steak in non-stick skillet; add water. Place in roasting pan with cover. Top with vegetables and water; sprinkle with spices. Cover and bake at 350 degrees for 1-1/2 hours. Serve over whole wheat noodles. Makes 4 servings; one serving counts as your protein and part of your simple carbohydrate.

*May use 2 large chicken breasts, deboned, skinned and split.

8) **EASY CHICKEN AND RICE** — (your protein, your complex carbohydrate and part of your simple
carbohydrate)
CAESAR SALAD — (your healthy munchie and added fat)
OR
PEACH PIZZAZZ — (this would be more simple carbohydrate)

EASY CHICKEN AND RICE — A great one dish meal

2 cups chicken stock, or low sodium chicken bouillon
3/4 cup water   **1/2 tsp. salt (optional)**
1 cup brown rice, uncooked   **1/4 tsp. black pepper**
4 boneless chicken breasts, skinned **1/2 tsp. garlic powder**
1 small onion, chopped   **1/2 tsp. rosemary**
1 Tbsp. dried parsley   **1 tsp. dried tarragon**
1 bag (16 oz.) frozen cuts of vegetables (i.e. California Mix)

Pour chicken stock and water into a large roasting pan. Add brown rice and top with chicken breasts. Sprinkle with chopped onion, herbs and spices. Cover pan with lid. Bake for 1-1/2 hours, adding the frozen vegetables during the last 30 minutes of cooking. This is a classic meal-in-one: 1 serving give 3 oz. protein, 2 complex carbohydrates and 1 simple carbohydrate.

CAESAR SALAD

4 cups washed, torn romaine	**1/8 tsp. salt (optional)**
1 clove minced garlic	**1 coddled egg***
1-1/2 Tbsp. olive oil	**juice of 1 lemon**
1/2 tsp. dry mustard	**1/4 cup grated parmesan**
1 tsp. worcestershire sauce	**1/8 tsp. coarse black pepper**

Croutons made from 2 slices whole wheat bread sprinkled with garlic powder, toasted till brown

Rub bottom and sides of large salad bowl with garlic; leave in bowl. Add oil, mustard, worcestershire sauce and spices; beat together with fork. Add chilled romaine lettuce; toss well. Top with coddled egg and lemon juice; toss till lettuce is well covered. Top with parmesan and croutons. Toss well and enjoy! Makes 6 servings. This gives a healthy munchie and an added fat.

*Coddle an egg by immersing the egg in shell in boiling water 30 seconds.

Our problem isn't not knowing what is right, it is doing it.

157

PEACH PIZZAZZ

4 peach halves, fresh or packed in own juice, without sugar
3 Tbsp. light or nonfat cream cheese
cinnamon

Place peach halves on lettuce leaves; top with 2 tsp. cheese and sprinkle with cinnamon. Makes 4 servings; each counts as simple carbohydrate.

The man who believes he can do something is probably right, and so is the man who believes he can't.

9) **SPAGHETTI PIE** — (your protein, complex carbohydrate and part of your simple carbohydrate)
MARINATED VEGGIES — (variety of raw veggies marinated in No-Oil Italian Dressing, sprinkled with Parmesan Cheese)

SPAGHETTI PIE

6 oz. Vermicelli or whole wheat pasta	**8 oz. can stewed tomatoes**
2 tsp. olive oil	**6 oz. can tomato paste**
1/3 cup grated Parmesan Cheese	**3/4 tsp. dried oregano**
2 egg whites, well beaten	**1/4 tsp. salt (optional)**
1/2 lb. ground turkey*	**1/2 tsp. garlic powder**
1/2 cup chopped onion	**1 cup part skimmed Ricotta Cheese**
1/4 cup chopped green pepper	**1/2 cup shredded Mozzarella Cheese**

Cook pasta according to package directions; drain. Stir olive oil and Parmesan Cheese into hot pasta. Add egg whites, stirring well. Spoon mixture into a 10" pie plate. Use a spoon to shape the spaghetti into a pie shell. Microwave at HIGH uncovered 3 minutes or until set. Set aside.

Crumble turkey in a colander, stir in onion and green pepper. Cover with plastic wrap and microwave at HIGH 5-6 minutes, stirring every 2 minutes. Let drain well. Put into a bowl and stir in tomatoes, tomato paste and seasonings. Cover and microwave at HIGH 3-1/2 to 4 minutes, stirring once. Set aside.

Spread Ricotta evenly over pie shell. Top with meat sauce. Cover with plastic wrap and microwave at HIGH 6 to 6-1/2 minutes; sprinkle with Mozzarella Cheese. Microwave uncovered at HIGH 30 seconds, or until cheese begins to melt.

6 servings = 2 oz. protein, 1 complex and 1 simple carbohydrate.

*May substitute ground round; drain well after cooking.

159

SURVIVAL PLANNING FOR QUICK MEALS

(This is for the people with the philosophy that
"If it takes longer to cook it than to eat it, FORGET IT!")

There are few pregnant moms with the time or inclination to spend all afternoon preparing the dinner meal each day. Spending just an hour on a weekend to put together some of the basics will allow each night's meal to be a healthy delight with a minimum of effort.

BASIC GAME PLAN: (Do once a week)

1) Prepare the marinade for Hawaiian Chicken; marinade enough boneless chicken breasts for 2 meals: 1/2 can be sliced and used in stir-fry with vegetables one night - the other breasts can be put on the grill.

2) Cook a big pot of brown rice - it can be heated during the week as needed. Or measure it out in servings, freeze in Ziplock® bags and reheat in microwave or boiling water.

3) Cook a big pot of whole wheat pasta for quick heat-ups during the week.

4) Make a pot of tomato sauce - it can be tossed with pasta, used to make "pita pizza," used to make lasagna, or as topping for meats. You may also keep commercial sauce made without salt or sugar for extra ease.

5) Cook a pot of pinto beans: they can be used one night as beans and rice, another night pureed and used on warm tortillas with shredded lettuce, chopped tomatoes and picante sauce as bean burritos.

6) Cut up a plastic bag full of various vegetables: zucchini, broccoli, cauliflower, mushrooms, carrots, etc. Part may be marinated in low calorie Italian dressing for a quick salad - remaining may be used to steam or stir-fry.

7) For "extra quick" stir-fry - use frozen bags of assorted vegetable mixes. The vegetables are already cut and they can be fully cooked in 4 minutes! Bags of frozen peas can also be used for a quick complex carbohydrate.

8) A basic salad is torn romaine lettuce topped with a tomato, a no-oil Italian dressing and a sprinkle of parmesan.

9) Sliced melon or fresh strawberries are a refreshing and quick complement to any meal!

A WEEK OF FAST AND FABULOUS DINNERS

Monday:
Grilled Marinated Chicken Breast
Brown Rice
Steamed Vegetables
Romaine Lettuce Salad

Tuesday:
Whole Wheat Pasta Topped with Tomato Sauce
  and Parmesan Cheese
Steamed Broccoli
Marinated Vegetables
Fresh Fruit Medley Topped with Yogurt

Wednesday:
Stir-fried Vegetables and Chicken Tossed with Pasta
Romaine Lettuce Salad

Thursday:
Beans over Brown Rice
Steamed Vegetables
Fresh Fruit

Friday:
Grilled Chicken on Whole Wheat Bun
Lettuce and Tomato Slices
Marinated Vegetable Salad

Saturday:
GO OUT TO EAT (or use up any leftovers)

Sunday:
Bean Burritos
Sliced Melon

162

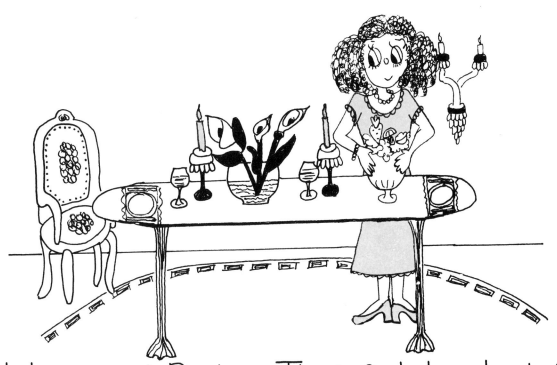

Holidays and Parties That Celebrate Life

HOLIDAYS AND PARTIES THAT CELEBRATE LIFE!

Here are survival tips for remaining alive, well and merry in a world that overeats: HAPPY HOLIDAYS!

1.   Always eat a healthy snack before going to parties so that your "appetite for the appetizers" will be in control!

2.   Don't try to starve the day of a big party! You will only slow down your metabolism and set yourself up for a gorge because you will be so hungry. Instead, eat smaller, evenly spaced meals throughout the day.

3.   Remember that it's not the "big parties" that are a problem - but the day by day eating. Eating well in between the "big days" will help to stabilize your body. Avoid the "I've blown it now" syndrome and let each day be a new beginning.

4.   Try to make the focus of parties more than just the food itself. Plan other activities besides eating! Games are fun for everyone and give a new direction from the usual gorge. Talk to friends in rooms other than where the food is served.

5.   Never tell people you are dieting; it is self sabotage! You will instantly be a candidate to be talked (or badgered!) into everything. If you feel you must say anything, just say "I am not hungry quite yet." Don't look pitiful in a corner! No one ever notices that the life of the party isn't eating.

RECIPES FOR WONDERFULLY HEALTHY HOLIDAYS
BEST BARBECUE

Date-Cheese Ball   Raw Vegetable Platter with Dips

Hawaiian Chicken *

Corn on the Cob   Cole Slaw with a Difference

Watermelon Quarters   Date Bars

DATE-CHEESE BALL

2 8 oz. pkgs. fat-free cream cheese	8 oz. chopped dates (not sugar-coated)
2 Tbsp. (or more) low-fat milk	1/2 cup chopped walnuts

Process in food processor or blender until evenly mixed. Use milk to help blend more easily. Shape into ball - garnish with grapes and walnuts. Best served with Norwegian Flat Breads. 2 Tbsp. = 1 protein and 1 simple carbohydrate.

ZESTY DIP

8 oz. low-fat cottage cheese	1/2 tsp. garlic powder
1 Tbsp. lemon juice	1/8 tsp. onion powder
2 tsp. celery seeds	1/4 tsp. salt (optional)
1 tsp. worcestershire sauce	dash red pepper sauce

Combine all ingredients in blender or processor. Process until cheese is consistency of sour cream. Serve with fresh vegetables for dipping. 1/4 cup gives 1 oz. protein.

* See index.

HERB AND GARLIC DIP

1 cup low-fat cottage cheese
1/2 cup skim milk
2 Tbsp. fresh or 1 Tbsp. dried parsley
1 small red cabbage

1/8 tsp. curry powder
1/8 tsp. paprika
1 garlic clove
1/2 tsp. basil

Place cottage cheese, milk, spices and garlic in blender or food processor, process until smooth. Hollow out the head of cabbage from the top. Cut a slice from the stem end so the cabbage will rest firmly on its base. Spoon dip into cabbage. 1/4 cup gives 1 oz. protein

COLE SLAW WITH A DIFFERENCE

1/4 head of red cabbage
1/4 head of green cabbage
2 large carrots

8 oz. crushed unsweetened pineapple
1/2 cup plain nonfat yogurt
1/2 cup raisins

Grate cabbage and carrots in food processor or by hand. Mix rest of ingredients together. This may be made far in advance — the flavors blend together. Makes 8 servings, each equaling 1 simple carbohydrate.

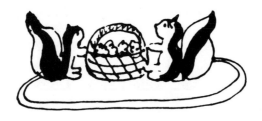

DATE BARS

1 cup whole wheat pastry flour	1 cup dates, chopped
1/2 cup wheat germ	1/2 cup chopped walnuts
1 tsp. baking powder	3 eggs, beaten
2 tsp. cinnamon	1/3 cup honey
1/4 tsp. ground allspice	1 tsp. vanilla extract

Combine the flour, wheat germ, baking powder, cinnamon, allspice, dates and walnuts in a medium mixing bowl. Mix the eggs, honey and vanilla together in a medium bowl, then fold into the dry ingredients. Spread the batter in a lightly oiled 9 x 13 inch baking pan. Bake at 350 degrees for about 20 minutes, until golden brown. Makes 24 bars, 2 bars equals 1 complex and 1 simple carbohydrate and 1 added fat.

The best way to keep children home is to make the home atmosphere pleasant - and let the air out of the tires.

167

HOLIDAY DINNER

Cranberry Salad Mold
Roast Turkey or Rosemary Roast Lamb
Wild Rice Pilaf*   Healthy Gravy
Sweet Potatoes Glorious   Green Beans with Mushrooms*
Apple-Date Muffins   Fresh Fruit Pie

CRANBERRY SALAD MOLD

2 envelopes unflavored gelatin
1 cup orange juice
1 - 6 oz. can apple juice concentrate
2 tbsp. honey
1 cup water

1 - 12 oz. bag cranberries
1 cup shredded carrot
1/2 cup raisins
1 cup chopped apple
1 cup diced celery

Sprinkle gelatin over juices and honey in small bowl, let soften 5 minutes. Meanwhile, combine cranberries and water in large saucepan. Bring to boiling. Lower heat and simmer 5 minutes. Add gelatin-juice mixture to cranberries. Stir until gelatin is dissolved, about 2 minutes. Let cool in refrigerator until thickened to consistency of egg whites. Add celery, carrot, raisins and apple; gently mix. Pour into a 6-cup mold that has been sprayed with non-stick cooking spray. Refrigerate overnight or until salad is firm. Makes 12 servings each counting as 2 simple carbohydrates.

*See index

ROAST TURKEY

Before roasting, slide a thin layer of celery leaves and thin slices of onion between skin and breast meat of turkey - it adds a rich flavor to the meat and the vegetables absorb much of the fat from the skin. Roast the turkey as you usually would.

TURKEY GRAVY — THE HEALTHY WAY

2 Tbsp. canola oil
1 Tbsp. cornstarch
1 bay leaf
1/4 cup white wine

1 clove minced garlic
1-1/2 cups heated chicken/turkey stock
(may use low sodium boullion)

Heat oil in saucepan. Add garlic and cook about 30 seconds. Stir in cornstarch until smooth. Add stock, bay leaf and wine. Cook until sauce thickens, about 5 minutes. Remove bay leaf. Serve with turkey. Makes about 2 cups. Each 1/3 cup serving equals 1 added fat.

ROSEMARY ROAST LAMB

6-7 lbs. oven-ready leg of lamb, trimmed of all visible fat
2 sliced garlic cloves
1 tsp. olive oil
2 tsp. rosemary
1/2 tsp. each salt and pepper
1 lb. green beans, boiled 5 minutes
**   and drained**
1 lb. can tomatoes, drained

1 lb. eggplant, halved crosswise
**   and cut into 1" spears**
1 lb. Idaho potatoes in 1" chunks
1 cup chicken broth
1/2 tsp. garlic powder
2-1/2 cups sliced onions

Heat oven to 400 degrees. With sharp knife make 6 small incisions in thickest part of meat and insert garlic slices. Rub meat with olive oil; sprinkle with rosemary and 1/2 tsp. each salt and pepper; press seasonings into meat. Put meat in large roasting pan and roast 1 hour and 15 minutes. Surround meat with vegetables, making two piles of each. Pour chicken broth over vegetables, making two piles of each. Pour chicken broth over vegetables and sprinkle with garlic powder, onions, tomatoes. Cover the pan with aluminum foil and bake 1 hour and 10 minutes more. Meat will be medium-rare to medium and internal temperature will register 150 degrees on a meat thermometer. Arrange sliced meat on platter surrounded with vegetables. 8 servings; each gives 3 oz. protein, 1 complex carbohydrate and 1 simple carbohydrate.

170

SWEET POTATOES GLORIOUS

4 lbs. sweet potatoes, boiled and peeled
2 Tbsp. cornstarch
1/2 tsp. salt (optional)
1-1/3 cups pineapple juice
1 small can crushed unsweetened pineapple

2 Tbsp. dry milk
3 eggs
1/2 tsp. cinnamon
2 tsp. nutmeg

Mash potatoes. Add all but pineapple — beat. Add pineapple and pour into casserole dish. Sprinkle with shredded coconut and walnuts as garnish. Bake at 350 degrees for 30 minutes. Freezes beautifully. 1/3 cup equals 1 complex CHO.

God sends food for the birds but He doesn't throw it in the nest.

APPLE DATE MUFFINS - Delicious!

1-1/2 cups Shredded Wheat-N-Bran cereal
1-1/2 cups whole wheat pastry flour
1 Tbsp. baking powder
1/2 tsp. salt (optional)
1/2 tsp. each cinnamon and apple pie spice
2 Tbsp. Canola oil

1/4 cup honey
1 cup skim milk
2 eggs
1/2 cup walnuts
1 cup dates, chopped
3 cups chopped apples

Finely process cereal in blender or food processor. Mix with remaining dry ingredients; set aside. In another bowl, beat oil, honey and eggs until well blended. Add skim milk. Stir in flour mixture till well blended; fold in dates and nuts. Spray muffin tin with non-stick cooking spray or line with papers; fill 2/3 full. Sprinkle top with dash of cinnamon. Bake at 350 degrees for 25 minutes or until toothpick inserted in center comes out clean. Cool on wire rack for 10 minutes; remove from pan and cool completely. Makes 16 muffins, each giving a complex CHO, 1 simple CHO and 1 added fat.

FRESH FRUIT PIE

1 cup unsweetened* flaked coconut   **2 egg whites, lightly beaten**

Toss together and pat into pie pan. Bake at 325 degrees for 10 minutes; cool.

Layer into shell:
2 bananas, sliced in orange juice and drained
1 pt. fresh sliced strawberries (or substitute sliced Kiwi)
15-1/2 oz. can of crushed unsweetened pineapple, cooked with 1 tsp. corn-starch to thicken

Sprinkle with more coconut and strawberries to garnish. Makes 8 servings, each equals 1 simple carbohydrate and 1 added fat.

*Available from natural food store

We always have time for the things we put first.

173

RECIPE INDEX AND NUTRITIONAL PROFILE

APPLE DATE MUFFINS, Page 172
Calories: 157; carbohydrate: 27 gm; protein: 4 gm; fat: 2 gm; calories from fat: 23%; cholesterol: 0 mg; sodium: 85 mg

CAESAR SALAD, Page 157
Calories: 81; carbohydrate: 6 gm; protein: 4 gm; fat: 5 gm; calories from fat: 51%; cholesterol: 39 mg; sodium: 152 mg

CARROT-CHEESE MELT, Page 143
Calories: 361; carbohydrate: 45 gm; protein: 25 gm; fat: 9 gm; calories from fat: 22%; cholesterol: 24 mg; sodium: 578 mg

CARROT SALAD, Page 145
Calories: 62; carbohydrate: 14 gm; protein: 2 gm; fat: 0 gm; calories from fat: 0%; cholesterol: 0 mg; sodium: 28 mg

CEREAL, (PERFECT BOWL OF), Page 138
Calories: 319; carbohydrate: 68 gm; protein: 14 gm; fat: 1 gm; calories from fat: 3%; cholesterol: 4 mg; sodium: 426 mg

CHEESE APPLE SURPRISE, Page 139
Calories: 332; carbohydrate: 41 gm; protein: 19 gm; fat: 11 gm; calories from fat: 30%; cholesterol: 32 mg; sodium: 586 mg

CHEESE DANISH, Page 135
USING FAT FREE CREAM CHEESE: Calories: 249; carbohydrate: 48 gm; protein: 12 gm; fat: 1 gm; calories from fat: 0%; cholesterol: 10 mg; sodium: 736 mg

USING LIGHT CREAM CHEESE: Calories: 328; carbohydrate: 48 gm; protein: 12 gm; fat: 11 gm; calories from fat: 30%; cholesterol: 48 mg; sodium: 736 mg

CHEF'S SALAD, Page 141
(without dressing) Calories: 285; carbohydrate: 24 gm; protein: 30 gm; fat: 7 gm; calories from fat: 23%; cholesterol: 61 mg; sodium: 442 mg

CHICKEN AND RICE, Page 156
Calories: 369; carbohydrate: 42 gm; protein: 27 gm; fat: 7 gm; calories from fat: 18%; cholesterol: 70 mg; sodium: 292 mg

CHICKEN, BASQUE, Page 153
WHOLE MEAL: Calories: 408; carbohydrate: 59 gm; protein: 33 gm; fat: 4 gm; calories from fat: 8%; cholesterol: 73 mg; sodium: 103 mg

CHICKEN, HAWAIIAN, Page 147
Calories: 182; carbohydrate: 5 gm; protein: 27 gm; fat: 3 gm; calories from fat: 16%; cholesterol: 72 mg; sodium: 126 mg

CHICKEN, OF THE LAND OR SEA SANDWICH, Page 142
Calories: 233; carbohydrate: 16 gm; protein: 25 gm; fat: 8 gm; calories from fat: 30%; cholesterol: 40 mg; sodium: 650 mg

CHICKEN, OVEN BAKED, Page 144
Calories: 176; carbohydrate: 7 gm; protein: 27 gm; fat: 4 gm; calories from fat: 21%; cholesterol: 108 mg; sodium: 123 mg

CHICKEN, STIR-FRY, Page 154
Calories: 235; carbohydrate: 15 gm; protein: 28 gm; fat: 7 gm; calories from fat: 27%; cholesterol: 72 mg; sodium: 126 mg

CHILI, CON CARNE, Page 152
Calories: 274; carbohydrate: 24 gm; protein: 21 gm; fat: 8 gm; calories from fat: 28%; cholesterol: 47 mg; sodium: 545 mg

COLE SLAW WITH A DIFFERENCE, Page 166
Calories: 58; carbohydrate: 13 gm; protein: 1 gm; fat: 0 gm; calories from fat: 0%; cholesterol: 0 mg; sodium: 20 mg

CRANBERRY SALAD MOLD, Page 168
Calories: 84; carbohydrate: 21 gm; protein: 0 gm; fat: 0 gm; calories from fat: 0%; cholesterol: 0 mg; sodium: 15 mg

DATE BARS, Page 167
Calories: 155; carbohydrate: 29 gm; protein: 4 gm; fat: 3 gm; calories from fat: 20%; cholesterol: 0 mg; sodium: 2 mg

DATE CHEESE BALL, Page 165
Calories: 51; carbohydrate: 7 gm; protein: 3 gm; fat: 1 gm; calories from fat: 18%; cholesterol: 0 mg; sodium: 71 mg

DIP, HERB AND GARLIC, Page 166
2 TBSP.: Calories: 20; carbohydrate: 1 gm; protein: 4 gm; fat: 0 gm; calories from fat: 0%; cholesterol: 1 mg; sodium: 122 mg

DIP, ZESTY, Page 165
2 TBSP.: Calories: 16; carbohydrate: 1 gm; protein: 3 gm; fat: 0 gm; calories from fat: 0%; cholesterol: 1 mg; sodium: 120 mg

FRESH FRUIT PIE, Page 173
Calories: 99; carbohydrate: 17 gm; protein: 1 gm; fat: 3 gm; calories from fat: 27%; cholesterol: 0 mg; sodium: 2 mg

FRENCH TOAST, Page 137
Calories: 329; carbohydrate: 55 gm; protein: 20 gm; fat: 3 gm; calories from fat: 7%; cholesterol: 3 mg; sodium: 529 mg

GRAVY, HEALTHFUL, Page 169
    Calories: 40; carbohydrate: 0 gm; protein: 0 gm; fat: 4.5 gm; calories from fat: all;
    cholesterol: 0 mg; sodium: 10 mg

GREEN BEANS AND MUSHROOMS, Page 129
    Calories: 52; carbohydrate: 9 gm; protein: 2 gm; fat: 2 gm; calories from fat: 17%;
    cholesterol: 0 mg; sodium: 4 mg

GREEN BEANS, COLORFUL, Page 148
    Calories: 53; carbohydrate: 9 gm; protein: 2 gm; fat: 1 gm; calories from fat: 17%;
    cholesterol: 0 mg; sodium: 4 mg

HAMBURGER, HEALTHY, Page 143
    (without condiments) Calories: 261; carbohydrate: 29 gm; protein: 22 gm; fat: 6 gm;
    calories from fat: 21%; cholesterol: 42 mg; sodium: 424 mg

LAMB, ROSEMARY ROAST, Page 170
    Calories: 254; carbohydrate: 26 gm; protein: 24 gm; fat: 7 gm; calories from fat:
    23%; cholesterol: 63 mg; sodium: 281 mg

MEATLOAF, MARVELOUS, Page 146
    Calories: 213; carbohydrate: 11 gm; protein: 22 gm; fat: 9 gm; calories from fat:
    25%; cholesterol: 98 mg; sodium: 257 mg

MUFFINS, APPLE DATE, Page 172
    Calories: 157; carbohydrate: 27 gm; protein: 4 gm; fat: 4 gm; calories from fat: 23%;
    cholesterol: 0 mg; sodium: 85 mg

OATMEAL WITH A DIFFERENCE, Page 136
    Calories: 357; carbohydrate: 63 gm; protein: 17 gm; fat: 4 gm; calories from fat:
    10%; cholesterol: 4 mg; sodium: 131 mg

PARFAIT, BREAKFAST, Page 139
Calories: 394; carbohydrate: 80 gm; protein: 20 gm; fat: 1 gm; calories from fat: 2%; cholesterol: 4 mg; sodium: 573 mg

PIZZAZZ, PEACH, Page 158
Calories: 28; carbohydrate: 7 gm; protein: less than 1 gm; fat: 0 gm; calories from fat: 0%; cholesterol: 0 mg; sodium: 5 mg

PEANUT BUTTER AND BANANA SANDWICH, Page 140
Calories: 346; carbohydrate: 52 gm; protein: 15; fat: 9 gm; calories from fat: 23%; cholesterol: 3 mg; sodium: 378 mg

PEANUT BUTTER DANISH, Page 136
Calories: 374; carbohydrate: 53 gm; protein: 18; fat: 10 gm; calories from fat: 25%; cholesterol: 4 mg; sodium: 418 mg

PEAS, ROSEMARY, Page 145
Calories: 83; carbohydrate: 12 gm; protein: 4 gm; fat: 2 gm; calories from fat: 23%; cholesterol: 0 mg; sodium: 95 mg

SALMON, BAKED IN A POUCH, Page 149
Calories: 168; carbohydrate: 3 gm; protein: 23 gm; fat: 5 gm; calories from fat: 27%; cholesterol: 42 mg; sodium: 62 mg

SALMON, GRILLED, Page 150
Calories: 157; carbohydrate: 0 gm; protein: 23 gm; fat: 5 gm; calories from fat: 29%; cholesterol: 42 mg; sodium: 50 mg

SALMON, LOAF, Page 151
Calories: 207; carbohydrate: 13 gm; protein: 22 gm; fat: 7 gm; calories from fat: 30%; cholesterol: 72 mg; sodium: 470 mg

SALMON, POACHED, Page 150
Calories: 161; carbohydrate: 1 gm; protein: 23 gm; fat: 5 gm; calories from fat: 28%; cholesterol: 42 mg; sodium: 62 mg

SANDWICH, CLASSIC, Page 141
Calories: 285; carbohydrate: 24 gm; protein: 30 gm; fat: 7 gm; calories from fat: 23%; cholesterol: 61 mg; sodium: 442 mg

SEAFOOD, SALAD, Page 140
WHOLE MEAL: Calories: 233; carbohydrate: 16 gm; protein: 25 gm; fat: 8 gm; calories from fat: 30%; cholesterol: 40 mg; sodium: 650 mg

SHAKE, BREAKFAST, Page 138
Calories: 200; carbohydrate: 32 gm; protein: 16 gm; fat: 2 gm; calories from fat: 10%; cholesterol: 5 mg; sodium: 176 mg

SPAGHETTI PIE, Page 159
Calories: 248; carbohydrate: 21 gm; protein: 23 gm; fat: 8 gm; calories from fat: 29%; cholesterol: 46 mg; sodium: 349 mg

SPINACH AND APPLE SALAD, Page 155
Calories: 69; carbohydrate: 12 gm; protein: 1 gm; fat: 2 gm; calories from fat: 26%; cholesterol: 0 mg; sodium: 30 mg

STEAK, ITALIAN SWISS, Page 155
Calories: 345; carbohydrate: 35 gm; protein: 35 gm; fat: 6.5 gm; calories from fat: 17%; cholesterol: 71 mg; sodium: 71 mg

SWEET POTATOES GLORIOUS, Page 171
Calories: 82; carbohydrate: 18 gm; protein: 2 gm; fat: 0 gm; calories from fat: 22%; cholesterol: 21 mg; sodium: 15 mg

VEGGIES, MARINATED, Page 159
  Calories: 67; carbohydrate: 8 gm; protein: 2 gm; fat: 3 gm; calories from fat: 40%; cholesterol: 0 mg; sodium: 340 mg

VEGGIE SANDWICH, Page 142
  WITH LEAN AND FREE CHEESE: Calories: 233; carbohydrate: 31 gm; protein: 25 gm; fat: 1 gm; calories from fat: 4%; cholesterol: 32 mg; sodium: 712 mg

WALDORF IN DISGUISE SALAD, Page 151
  Calories: 114; carbohydrate: 22 gm; protein: 2 gm; fat: 2 gm; calories from fat: 18%; cholesterol: 0 mg; sodium: 53 mg

WILD RICE PILAF, Page 148
  Calories: 122; carbohydrate: 21 gm; protein: 4 gm; fat: 2 gm; calories from fat: 22%; cholesterol: 0 mg; sodium: 210 mg

LOOK FOR THESE OTHER BOOKS BY CAROLYN COATS AND PAMELA SMITH

Things Your Mother Always Told You But You Didn't Want to Hear
Warm, witty, nostalgic words of wisdom you'll remember forever with love.
ISBN 0-7852-8056-1

Things Your Dad Always Told You But You Didn't Want to Hear
Funny, profound, memorable. The perfect companion to the "Mother" book. Great for men's and boys' birthday gifts.
ISBN 0-7852-8055-3

My Grandmother Always Said That
From generation to generation, grandmothers have always said the same wise words to their families. They do it because they love them, but mostly because they just can't help it.
ISBN 0-7852-8053-7

Me, A Gourmet Cook?
A delightful cookbook full of easy but delicious recipes and creative, entertaining ideas. Perfect for graduation and new brides and grooms.
ISBN 0-7852-8052-9

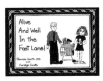

Alive and Well in the Fast Lane
The very latest information on how to lower your cholesterol and risk of cancer; how to increase your energy and stamina and achieve your ideal weight. The 10 Commandments of good nutrition plus great recipes and tips.
ISBN 0-7852-8050-2

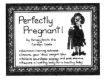

Perfectly Pregnant!
The latest information to perfectly nourish you and your baby —hints to overcome morning sickness, assure ideal weight gain, and maintain your energy and stamina. The perfect gift for that "special lady."
ISBN 0-7852-8054-5

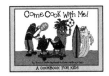

Come Cook With Me!
Shhh . . . Don't tell the kids, but this wonderful book has recipes that are delicious, fun to make AND nutritious. The gift every grandmother and parent will love to give.
ISBN 0-7852-8051-0

Available at fine bookstores everywhere.
THOMAS NELSON PUBLISHERS
Nashville, Tennessee 37214

OTHER BOOKS AND TAPES
BY PAMELA M. SMITH, R.D.

Eat Well - Live Well

The nutrition guide and cookbook for healthy, productive people. This large, hardback edition presents "The Ten Commandments of Good Nutrition" in detail, cooking tips, menu planning, grocery shopping, a dining-out guide and a large cookbook section of innovative recipes that can be prepared in a time-saving manner. Meal plans are also included.

The Food Trap

As she explores our relationship with food, Pamela Smith asks, *Is the refrigerator light the light of your life?* Informative and enlightening, this book reveals case studies and personal insights into the physical, emotional, and spiritual aspects of food dependencies. Learn how to break free in all areas.

The Food Trap Seminar

In this audio tape album from a live seminar, Pamela Smith discusses our physical, emotional, and spiritual needs and how to meet and nourish these needs properly. She also presents a nutritional strategy for dealing with stress. Very practical and informative.

Free Tape Offer

For a free audio-cassette tape on nutrition principles by Pamela Smith, please complete and mail the following coupon (plus U.S. $2.00 to cover postage and handling).

Please send me a free copy of "Nutrition Principles" Audio Tape
by Pamela Smith.
I have enclosed U.S. $2.00 to cover postage and handling.

Name:_____

Address:_____

City: _____ State: _____ Zip Code:_____

Send coupon and money to:
Pamela M. Smith, R.D. • P.O. Box 541009 • Orlando, FL 32854

Published in Nashville, Tennessee, by Thomas Nelson, Inc., Publishers, and distributed in Canada by Word Communications, Ltd., Richmond, British Columbia, and in the United Kingdom by Word (UK), Ltd., Milton Keynes, England.

Library of Congress information

Smith, Pamela M.
How to be perfectly pregnant! / by Pamela Smith and Carolyn Coats.
    p.   cm.
"Revised 1993."
Cover title: Perfectly pregnant.
Originally published: Orlando, Fla. : Carolyn Coats' Bestsellers, 1988.
Includes index.
ISBN: 0-7852-8054-5
1. Pregnancy—Nutritional aspects. 2. Cookery. I. Coats, Carolyn, 1935- . II. Title. III. Title: Perfectly pregnant.
RG559.S65 1994
618.2'4—dc20
                                                                                        93-43102
                                                                                        CIP

Printed in the United States of America

1 2 3 4 5 6 7 - 99 98 97 96 95 94